CONQUERING COMPULSIVE EATING

CONQUERING COMPULSIVE EATING

A complete self-help guide

Alice Katz, M.S.

International Self-Counsel Press Ltd.
Head and Editorial Office
Vancouver
Toronto   Seattle

Printed in Canada

Printed in Canada.

First edition: October, 1986

Katz, Alice, 1935-
    Conquering compulsive eating

    (Self-counsel series)
    ISBN 0-88908-637-0

    1. Reducing — Psychological aspects. I. Title. II. Series.
    RC552.A72K38 1986   613.2'5'019   C86-091373-2

Cover design by Sara Woodwark

Cover props courtesy of Mozart Tearoom & Restaurant, 1011 Robson Street,
Vancouver, B.C.

SELF-COUNSEL SERIES

International Self-Counsel Press Ltd.
Editorial Office
306 West 25th Street
North Vancouver
British Columbia   V7N 2G1
Canada

Self-Counsel Press Inc.
1303 N. Northgate Way
Seattle
Washington, 98133 U.S.A.
*(a subsidiary of International
Self-Counsel Press Ltd.)*

CONTENTS

LIST OF EXERCISES

LIST OF CHARTS

PREFACE

If you are now a compulsive eater, you can learn to have a life minus compulsive eating by changing your beliefs about food, about feelings, and about being fat. By recognizing that the ideas you have are irrational, you can gradually replace them with more realistic and objective ones.

This book is based on the concept that your thoughts create your feelings, which for the compulsive eater are almost always unhappy. To cope, the compulsive eater uses food for comfort, reward, or distraction. You may realize, for example, that you are often upset, and you may blame your eating on that. If, however, you accept the idea that *you* are the source of your unhappiness because of the way you *think* about your life and yourself, and that it is your mind that triggers your eating, then you can see that by changing those thoughts, you will be less upset. You will then have much less need to use food to cope with negative feelings.

This book, then, is not about dieting to lose weight. It is, rather, a journey into your mind. It is intended to make you more aware of the messages you are giving yourself and where those messages originated. Do they make sense at this point in your life, if, indeed, they ever did?

Most of the concepts in this book are based on the work done with hundreds of men and women who sought counseling from The AL/CE Program for compulsive eating. It was only when these men and women took the mental journey that they were able to make significant changes in their eating and their lifestyles.

As you read this book, you can help yourself further by doing the exercises, keeping a journal of your feelings and behavior, reading other related material, and not judging yourself. You might also want to seek counseling or join a group that specializes in dealing with the emotional basis of compulsive eating.

1

WHAT IS COMPULSIVE EATING?

a. EATING AS A COMPULSIVE BEHAVIOR

Compulsive eating is just one type of addictive behavior. Alcoholism, drug abuse, smoking, and caffeine use are other common addictions. Both psychological and chemical factors contribute to them. Using these substances triggers a physical desire for more, and overuse leads to physical dependency.

Some compulsive behaviors have a psychological basis only. For example, compulsive spenders buy on impulse and cannot save their money. Compulsive gamblers don't stop when they run out of money; they may steal to continue. Compulsive cleaners become upset by any disarray and spend hours keeping everything in order. Compulsive savers never throw anything out.

Both psychological and chemical factors contribute to compulsive eating behavior. When you eat *some* chocolate, caffeine, or sugar your body needs more. Sugar and carbohydrates elevate your blood sugar level; when that level drops, your body needs more to elevate it again.

However, despite the chemical factors that complicate compulsive eating, this behavior is primarily a psychological problem. *Compulsive eating is any eating done in response to your mind instead of your body.* Your body will respond to hunger and internal cues, but when you eat beyond the point of satisfaction, it is your *mind* that keeps you going. When the contributing psychological factors are very strong, even the knowledge that a certain food is harmful may not be enough to prevent your eating. Since total abstinence from food is impossible, compulsive eating is the most difficult addiction to overcome.

Compulsive eating has several things in common with other addictions:

(a) It involves much of your time to the exclusion of many other things.

(b) It occupies your thoughts, even when you are not doing it.

(c) It cannot be given up unless you have help.

(d) Giving it up usually leaves you with withdrawal symptoms.

An addiction, in a sense, controls you, which means that you have no choice about it. But in another sense, you have made a choice. Because you derive some benefits from doing what you do, you choose to keep doing it.

1

The "benefits" gained from compulsive behavior include such things as:

(a) Time spent obsessing about the addiction leaves less time to think and worry about things that cause anxiety.

(b) The addiction provides a diversion from unpleasant chores like laundry or term papers.

(c) It removes you from reality and leaves you in a stupor, so you can blot out anxiety. This is especially true about alcohol, drugs, and sugar, but even excessive cleaning can do this.

(d) It gives you a temporary high, a kind of euphoria, until guilt sets in about what you did. Food does this when you feel full; gambling and spending money give a sense of danger and power.

(e) It brings a sense of order to your outer world, which you need if your inner world is chaotic. This refers especially to compulsive neatness.

These benefits are not usually recognized or acknowledged consciously, but they may be powerful enough to hinder change.

Eating compulsively is a way of indirectly taking care of emotional needs. It may result in unhappiness about weight or control, but unless your needs are met directly, the alternatives to eating may seem worse to you.

The negative consequences alone are not severe enough to stop the behavior. As an addiction, compulsive eating is probably the least harmful. It usually affects your health less than other forms of substance abuse, and any effects on your appearance are usually based on distorted ideas about beauty and its importance.

b. WHAT TRIGGERS COMPULSIVE EATING?

The desire to eat is triggered by hunger — a physical sensation. But *compulsive* eating is triggered by signals in your mind, not your stomach. If this happens too often, you lose touch with your normal body signals.

Some of the triggers for compulsive eating are:

- *Food:* seeing it on a plate, in the market, in the refrigerator, in a pot, at a buffet, in an ad, on television. When you see it, you think, "It is there, so I must have it."
- *Time:* eating by the clock, instead of when hungry. This starts with rigid scheduled feeding as a baby, followed by having to eat at set times in school and then at work. You look at the clock and determine if it is time to eat, ignoring your body signals.

- *Habit:* eating while watching television, reading, riding in the car, or cooking. Snacking in front of the TV comes from years of buying popcorn and candy at the movies. As a child, you may have been given food in the car to keep you quiet. Now, you eat when you drive.
- *Associations and memories:* being given ice cream as a child after a hospital stay, for a birthday, or as a reward for good behavior, or being given cookies when you cried may lead you to want them now. When you have them, they stir up fond memories.
- *Feelings:* being angry, lonely, tired, even happy can lead to eating if you think that food will make you feel happier or better.

c. KINDS OF COMPULSIVE EATERS

1. The anorexic

Anorexia is a prolonged, non-medical loss of appetite. It is the most severe of all eating disorders and the most difficult to treat because it involves many distortions, especially about body size. The anorexic usually denies that anything is wrong and does not seek help. Typically, anorexia strikes young females with some history of being overweight. They are obsessed with being thin at any price, but believe they are fat.

The anorexic looks starved. She does not allow herself pleasure from food or anything else. She thinks about food all the time, and about *not* eating. She tells herself she is full, when she really is starving. She believes that any eating will make her fat. She thinks eating is being weak and prides herself on her denial.

2. Borderline anorexic (anorectic thinker)

This person thinks eating is bad and eats only limited amounts. She may be normal weight, but thinks she is overweight. She has a distorted body image. This is much more common to females than males.

Anorexia as such is not dealt with in this book, although many of the principles in the second half of the book also apply to it.

3. The bulimic

Bulimia is massive overeating followed (usually) by self-induced vomiting. Many bulimics are former anorexics. As bulimics, they allow themselves to eat, but they binge as the result of having felt starved for so long. The binges are seen as a weakness, so they compensate by purging through vomiting or by using laxatives. Thus, the bulimic has devised a way to eat without guilt and without gaining weight.

3

In order to purge, the bulimic must consume huge quantities of food. This is done alone, so there is a secret quality to the eating and purging.

4. The bulimic thinker

The true bulimic binges and purges. The bulimic thinker is a binger-starver, following the same principles. At times, maybe once a week, or once a day, the binger-starvers eat to the point of discomfort, then regret it and either diet or fast. Binger-starvers shift between overeating and undereating. They have a distorted body image and see themselves as fat, but they are less secretive about what they do. If your weight yo-yos because you are always "on" or "off" a diet, you fit in this category.

5. The compulsive overeater

Overeaters eat too often or too long and weigh too much as a result. In time, they may become obese. The eating disorder, therefore, is apparent to others, unlike bulimia. Although overeaters claim they want to be thinner, they may have fears about being so. When they do stop overeating and lose weight, they often panic and go back to old habits.

d. ARE YOU A COMPULSIVE EATER?

Where do you fit in? Do you have some characteristics of all of the conditions described? Have you been different at different times? You can begin to make changes when you can see how you think and what you do. Use the checklist in Exercise #1 to quickly assess whether you are a compulsive eater.

EXERCISE #1
COMPULSIVE EATER CHECKLIST

☐	1.	I think about food much of the day.
☐	2.	I live to eat more than I eat to live.
☑	3.	I spend a lot of each day eating.
☑	4.	I eat when I am not hungry.
☐	5.	I never say no to an offer of food.
☑	6.	I feel controlled by food.
☑	7.	I get strong cravings for specific foods.
☑	8.	I eat when I get upset.
☐	9.	Eating makes me feel better.
☑	10.	I can only diet for short periods of time.

If you have checked five or more of the boxes, you are a compulsive eater. If you are, take heart that you are one of millions and that reading this book can help you.

2
PLANNING FOR CHANGE

a. CLARIFYING YOUR MOTIVES

Before you can begin to implement a program to overcome your overeating, you must understand *why* you want to change. Are you making assumptions about what your life will be like once you do conquer your overeating? Fill in the questionnaire in Exercise #2 before reading on.

EXERCISE #2
CLARIFYING GOALS

1. I am unhappy about being a compulsive eater because:
   a. _I don't look pretty_
   b. _I don't feel well_
   c. _It depresses me_

2. If I did not eat compulsively, then my life would change in these ways:
   a. _I would look and feel healthier_
   b. _I might attract men_
   c. _I would be more outgoing — more sure of myself._

3. Other people who are unhappy about my overeating are:
   a. _my mother_
   b. _my boss_

4. The times in my life when I have eaten most compulsively are when:
   a. _I am angry, hurt or depressed_
   b. _I am bored_

5. The times when I have been most successful at stopping my compulsive eating are when:
   a. _I am feeling good about myself_
   b. _I am busy_

Here are the most common reasons for wanting to stop overeating. Do these reasons correspond with your answers to the questionnaire?

- *You feel out of control.* Do you feel that you eat automatically, that there is no sense of choice about starting or stopping? Do you pride yourself on having control in most other areas?
- *You feel ashamed of the way you eat.* Do you think it is undignified, and do you label yourself a "pig" or "glutton?" Do you dislike yourself?
- *You feel uncomfortable.* Do you often feel tired and bloated?
- *You worry about your health.* Do you have medical problems such as edema, high blood pressure, or gallstones? Are you concerned about preventing future problems, such as diabetes, because of excess sugar and fatty foods?
- *You are overweight.* Are your clothes too tight? Do you dislike your appearance?
- *You have no time for other things.* Does food occupy all your time? Are you always thinking about not eating?
- *You are home too much.* Do you spend too much time alone because you are ashamed of your behavior or your appearance?
- *Your spouse or parent wants you to change (get thinner).* Do you feel pressured to change? (Unfortunately, this last reason will not motivate you to change, but, more likely, will cause you to feel resentment. Then, you will eat even more than usual out of spite. You cannot change unless *you* want to.)

Here are the most common beliefs about how your life will improve if you stop overeating and some comments on them.

- *You will be more in control.* Do you consider "normal" eating as being in control? Actually, in order to eat normally, you have to give up the control you now have over your body, and let your body dictate to you. Then you will eat when you are hungry and stop when the hunger is gone. Also, you need to be in control in other areas of your life, and that takes work.
- *You will enjoy life more.* It is true that when you are less obsessed with food and with being slim, you will have more time to enjoy life. It is also true that when you enjoy life more, you eat less.
- *You will be less lonely.* When you spend less time with food, you may feel better about your eating and your weight and so want to be with people. It is also true that overeating may be used as an excuse not to be with people when being with them is scary.

- *You will like yourself better.* You probably will feel better about yourself when you eat less and weigh less, but it is also true that when you like yourself more, you will eat less and weigh less.
- *You will feel better.* It is good not to overeat, but it is important to eat healthy foods. So you have to eat more normal amounts, but also make substitutions for empty or unhealthy calories.
- *You will be happy.* Happiness comes from within; it depends on a positive attitude. Weighing less does not guarantee happiness.

b. WHY NOT DIET?

The premise of this book is that what you do with food is a metaphor, that is, it is symbolic of the way you live your life and the way you deal with your emotions. Therefore, your overeating is a *symptom* of a problem, not the problem itself. Your weight is also a symptom.

When you go on a diet, you deal only with the symptom, but the cause of overweight is overeating. A diet may take away the overweight and, for a while, the overeating, but it still leaves the cause of the overeating.

Dieting won't work. In fact, dieting can *increase* your compulsive eating and weight. If you had been successful at dieting, you would not be reading this book. Here are some of the reasons dieting won't solve your problem.

- *Dieting makes you feel deprived.* As a result, you go off the diet and eat what you want.
- *Dieting causes resentment.* You feel like a child being told what to do, so you rebel and eat.
- *Dieting is rigid and unnatural.* It is too difficult to eat at set times and only set amounts and prescribed foods.
- *Dieting ignores body signals.* When you eat in a prescribed way, you have to tune out signals that you are hungry or full because they are contrary to the diet. When you ignore them too long, you soon are unable to recognize body signals.
- *Dieting is a compulsive behavior.* If you are a perfectionist at all, you probably demand of yourself that you diet "perfectly." Eating any food that is not on the diet leads you to become so angry with yourself that you give up dieting. So when you diet, you exchange one compulsive behavior for another.
- *Dieting makes you dependent.* Unless you create the diet by yourself for your particular needs, you are using a diet some authority devised. This implies that you do not know what is

best for your body and that you cannot trust your body to tell you when to eat and how much to eat.

- *Dieting makes foods evil.* A diet consists of a list of foods that are acceptable because they are lower in calories. Those not on the list are unacceptable. The implication is that only those on the list are "good" foods and that all others are "bad." Depending on the diet, foods such as carrots and potatoes can be good or bad. This is true for many other foods too: coffee, liquor, carbohydrates, protein. Whatever diet you are on, you believe in the intrinsic morality of those foods. It is human nature to want what is forbidden, so no one can diet for long.

- *Dieting can lead to increased weight.* When you lose weight, your metabolic rate decreases to compensate. When you go off a diet and increase your eating, your metabolism is no longer high enough to burn up the added calories without increased exercise. So, unless you do exercise, you gain again and the new weight stays. Over a period of years, your weight goes up instead of down from inconsistent dieting.

- *Dieting leads to compulsive eating.* For all of the above reasons, you are unable to diet for very long. When you do go off the diet, even if it is just by eating one food at one sitting, you feel so upset with yourself that you decide to eat even more. Or you feel so deprived or resentful from not eating what you want that the diet becomes a trigger to overeat.

c. THE CART BEFORE THE HORSE

Thinking that losing weight is the answer to all your problems is putting the cart before the horse. The same is true about giving up your compulsive eating. You may say you dislike yourself now because you are overweight and eat too much, but that when you eat normally and get thinner, you will feel good about yourself. You will socialize more, be more assertive, or express your feelings better.

Actually, the reverse is true. You eat because your self-image is poor and because of distortions and misconceptions you have about yourself and others. Overeating compounds the problem, and you feel worse when you are obsessed by weight and food.

You can see that there is a vicious circle between eating and self-image: when you don't like yourself, you overeat; when you overeat, you don't like yourself, etc.

When you increase your self-esteem, you decrease your overeating. But if you decrease your overeating only and your self-image remains the same, you will soon return to your pattern of overeating.

8

Overeating is actually a compensation for the things you feel lacking, and simply eating less or weighing less cannot change that.

d. STEPS TOWARD POSITIVE ACTION

When you know what factors contribute to your compulsive eating, you can begin to arrange your life so you will have consistent success in reducing it.

There are 10 strategies for change. If that seems like a lot, remember that they are all related to each other. Doing one will affect the others.

1. Gather information

You must understand what compulsive eating is and how you began. You have to look at what messages you were given as a child about food, about being thin, and about expressing feelings. You need to see how food was used when you were growing up.

2. Increase awareness

You need to make your eating less automatic by pinpointing what you eat, how much, when, what triggers it, and what foods you crave.

3. Know your motivation

You must know why you want to change.

4. Change habits

You must learn to replace junk foods with healthier ones, eat only what you love and desire, eat slowly, and eat only at a table.

5. Increase trust in your body

You must become more aware of when you are hungry and when you feel full and trust that if you listen to your body's signals you will weigh less.

6. Replace myths

You must get rid of misconceptions you have about food, feelings and fat, and replace them with more rational ideas.

7. Feed your emotional hunger

You need to identify your feelings and needs, and take care of them without using food to push them away.

8. Replace negative thinking

You need to increase your self-esteem and give yourself positive messages.

9. Take control
You must take control of your life by becoming assertive.

10. Take action
You must replace self-pity and feelings of hopelessness with *doing* and *expressing*, instead of *eating*.

3

UNDERSTANDING YOUR EATING PATTERNS

a. HOW YOU EAT

To overcome overeating, it is important to identify your particular style of overeating. That is the first step in turning an unconscious act into a conscious decision.

1. Eating styles

Look at the list of eating styles below. Which ones pertain to you?

(a) *The binger* eats normal amounts at meals, but eats great amounts at other times in one sitting, often late at night. Eating a lot at one sitting can be a reward for having been deprived all day of your favorite foods, especially if you eat very drab foods at meals. Your binge may be the result of not wanting to be seen indulging by others, so you may become a *sneak eater* who only binges when alone (see below).

(b) *The plate cleaner* eats until there is no more food on the plate or the table, regardless of appetite or capacity. Usually, plate cleaners were taught to always clean their plate as children, and this has become a habit that needs to be unlearned.

(c) *The nibbler* eats normal amounts at meals, but has countless mini-meals all day while doing other things such as cooking or talking on the phone. Nibblers fool themselves into thinking that they did not really eat much.

(d) *The snacker* eats normal amounts at meals, but eats many snacks — mostly junk food — between meals. Snackers may restrict what they eat at meals, and then feel deprived, so reward themselves by eating forbidden foods between meals. Snackers tend to convince themselves that the snacks do not count as calorie intake.

(e) *The stuffer* eats only at mealtimes, but always until really full and uncomfortable. If you are a stuffer, you have panicky feelings about being hungry, and so you overeat and never experience hunger. Or you may anticipate starting a diet tomorrow, so want to eat now while you can, like a camel storing water before a trek in the desert.

(f) *The stuffer-starver* feels guilty about overeating, so starves all day, feels very hungry at night, and eats until bedtime. The next day the cycle is repeated. When you behave this way, you feel deprived and overeat out of resentment.

(g) *The sneak eater* eats normal amounts or not at all in front of others; when alone, the sneak eater binges. Sneak eaters assume that their eating patterns matter to others, and so they pretend, by eating when they are alone, that they eat very little. They enjoy the secrecy involved.

(h) *The all-nighter* eats normal amounts during the day, then eats throughout the night, getting out of bed frequently to raid the refrigerator. It may be that this secret eating reflects a need for privacy; it may be the only thing in the all-nighter's life that is his or her own.

(i) *The comfort eater* eats normal amounts except when under stress, then eats until the anxiety is blotted out. Even small worries can trigger the eating. Comfort eaters have difficulty dealing with their feelings. They generally learned in childhood that it is better never to show feelings.

(j) *The gobbler* eats all food very fast, and as a result consumes more than if he or she had eaten slowly. People eat quickly either because they have an unconscious fear that they will not get their share or because they consider eating sinful and want to get it over with before they are caught. This may be your feeling even if you live alone and have no one watching you eat.

2. Your eating behavior profile

Do Exercise #3 now to determine your current eating patterns and how they are related to your past.

3. How to help yourself

The following suggestions apply to most of the eating styles discussed.

(a) Determine whether your eating behavior stems from messages learned as a child. If those messages no longer make sense, revise them. For instance, were you told to clean up your plate because there were "children starving in India?" Were you told that you could have dessert if you ate your vegetables? Do you do that now? Were you told never to waste food? These ingrained messages need not apply to your eating now. It is all right to throw out the food on your plate that you don't want. You do not need to eat it just because it is there. In fact, eating it may be wasteful if you then need to spend money on diet books and weight loss programs.

(b) See if your eating behavior now is the result of having the same attitudes you had as a child. For instance, were you

EXERCISE #3
YOUR EATING BEHAVIOR

Make a check mark next to every item that applies to you.

AS A CHILD

_____ I ate what I wanted.

_____ I was asked what I liked.

_____ I enjoyed eating.

_____ Mealtime was pleasant.

_____ I could leave food on the plate.

_____ Food was served in excess.

_____ No foods were forbidden.

✓ I had to eat what I was served.

_____ I was never asked what I liked.

✓ I was a picky eater.

✓ Mealtimes were tense.

_____ I had to finish every drop.

_____ Food was served sparingly.

_____ Sweets were forbidden.

✓ I ate in secret.

Some foods were forbidden

AS AN ADULT

✓ I eat foods I love.

_____ I only eat foods available.

_____ I only eat foods I should.

_____ I eat by the clock.

_____ I eat all the time.

_____ I eat only when I am hungry.

✓ I eat when I am upset.

✓ I eat at night.

_____ I eat when I see food.

_____ I eat only at the table.

_____ I eat at the stove.

✓ I eat while watching TV.

_____ I eat in the car.

✓ I eat in bed.

_____ I eat small meals at a time.

✓ I eat in binges.

_____ I binge, then starve.

_____ I binge, then purge.

✓ I starve all day, then eat all night.

✓ I eat for comfort.

_____ I eat to avoid chores.

✓ I eat to pass the time.

✓ I eat out of anger.

Compare the items checked for when you were a child to those you checked as an adult. Are there any similarities between your past and present relationship with food? List them below:

Eat in secret at night while going to bed

scolded for eating too much, so that now you never eat in front of others? Here are some other examples:

- You were not permitted to eat junk foods as a child, so now when you do, you hide it.
- Whenever you cried, you were given food, so now you comfort yourself the same way. It is an illusion to think that food can really give you comfort or solve your problems. The problems will be there when you stop eating.
- You come from a large family where there was never enough to eat, so now you panic about the next meal and stuff yourself so as not to get too hungry.

(c) Try to deal directly with your anger, so that if someone is telling you to eat less you can express your right to do what you want. Then you won't need to eat in secret.

(d) Establish your boundaries so that you have privacy. Then you need not seek privacy with food.

(e) Stop restricting what you eat; start eating the foods you love.

(f) Eat smaller meals and eat more frequently so you never get too hungry.

(g) Try to slow down your eating; time yourself and allow at least 20 minutes for a meal, or try eating with the wrong hand.

(h) Say no to an offer of food if you do not want it. You can do it politely and truthfully, saying you are too full.

These methods for helping yourself are discussed in greater detail in this chapter and later chapters.

b. WHAT YOU EAT

Your body is a machine like your car. Your stomach is the engine that needs fuel to run. That fuel is the food you put in it. It has a limited capacity of about two cups. Give it the wrong food, and your body breaks down, just as your car does if you put in the wrong gas. Underfill your stomach, and your body cannot work. Overfill it, and your body becomes sluggish.

How can you learn to make your health more important than the instant gratification of a binge? How can you learn to care about the ill effects of sugar more than the taste of candy now, especially if you have no adverse symptoms from eating it? How can you motivate yourself to eat less, or at least make healthier substitutions for some of the foods you now consume?

If you want to learn to eat healthy food now in order to prevent future ill health, you need to first learn to accept certain facts:

- You are worth being the best you can be, which means being healthy.
- You have some control over whether or not you are healthy.
- Your body wants to be healthy, and will fight any invasion of disease.
- It is more difficult for your body to struggle against disease when you are under stress.
- Your body can fight disease better with good nutrition.
- Environmental toxins and heredity will affect you less if you are healthy.

You have no control over your heredity and little over the environment. But you have a great deal of control over what you put into your body. To take care of the stress factor, you may need professional help. But since stress and disease are so closely linked, you can't ignore it.

What is your attitude about the health of your pets and your children? Are you very selective about what you feed your pet? If you have an infant, aren't you very careful about the foods you give him or her? If you have older children, do you think about the nutritional aspect of the meals you serve?

Why would you not treat yourself as well as you treat your loved ones? Why should you not care about your intake of sugar, salt, fat, and chemicals? Your body tells you when to eat and how much. WHAT you eat is up to you.

1. Foods as triggers

When you eat compulsively, you most likely always pick the same foods that seem to be triggers for all compulsive eaters: ice cream, candy, carbohydrates, and chocolate. Let us examine some of the reasons for this.

(a) Ice cream

There are many reasons why ice cream is so appealing: it is smooth and creamy and so goes down easily; when you are troubled, you want something soothing, that is, symbolically smooth with no rough edges. Metaphorically, ice cream fills the bill.

It is made from milk, which was the first food you had at the time when you were held by your mother. That was a time when you were free of worries and responsibilities. Milk combined with sugar makes ice cream: the food you associate with comfort.

Further, ice cream was probably given to you on special occasions, such as birthdays, so you associate it with pleasant memories. Those memories trigger you to eat the ice cream, especially when you are feeling down.

(b) Sweets

As a child, you were perhaps given dessert as a reward for finishing your meal. As an adult, you binge on sweets to reward yourself for eating healthy foods. Or, as a child, perhaps you were given cookies when you cried. As an adult, you binge on cookies whenever you are upset.

The sugar in cookies, cakes, and candies chemically triggers you to eat more by shooting insulin into your system, creating a "high" of energy, then dropping the blood sugar so that you need more to raise it. This is truer for some people than others; it is not as strong a trigger as the emotional ones.

(c) Carbohydrates

There is some evidence that you can be allergic to carbohydrates, such as cakes, breads, and pasta, and that you can crave those foods because they temporarily cause a reaction in your system.

You may also have emotional associations to some of these foods, such as the memory of freshly baked bread in the kitchen when you were a child.

(d) Chocolate

Chocolate contains a chemical to which you can become addicted.

If you had a lot of it as a child, you could have made eating it a habit, or it may evoke pleasant memories and be thought of as a reward food.

All sweets can symbolically represent "sweetening" your life, especially when you feel that it is full of misery.

2. Changing what you eat

There are several good reasons to change what you now eat:

(a) The foods you binge on are unhealthy and you worry about your health, especially if they contain sugar.

(b) The foods you binge on chemically trigger you to eat more of them, especially if they contain chocolate or sugar.

(c) You get very little pleasure from the food you now eat because you choose only what is good for you.

(d) You eat anything and never think about what you really want, and so get little pleasure from food.

None of these reasons has to do with losing weight. If your selection of food is based on losing weight rather than on personal preference, you will soon begin to binge on the foods you love. It is different if you create a diet for yourself including only foods you really like. Your choices may be in a form that is lower in calories, but it must be your choice and not someone else's.

The key to success is to REPLACE and SUBSTITUTE, not to give up what you like to eat.

3. Replacing foods

If you eat more of what you like to eat, you will eat less in total and lose weight. You can replace the unhealthy or fattening foods you now eat with foods that are just as tasty and satisfying, and you won't miss your old ones. The sections below discuss the foods that cause the most problems and suggest better replacements. The chart on page 19 provides a quick reference for you.

(a) Sugar

Most diets tell you to give up sweets. You try, but it doesn't work for very long because emotionally you crave a sweet as a treat for yourself. You probably know the harm sugar can cause your system: diabetes, hypoglycemia, tooth decay, depression. When you eliminate sugar from your diet, you immediately experience a clearer head and better spirits. For most compulsive sugar addicts, though, feeling better is not enough motivation to stop eating sweets. Therefore, you have to consider what to replace them with.

- Try sugarless cookies from a health food store. They will seem bitter until you cut out all sugar. Eat slowly and without guilt, and you will find you eat just a few.
- Eat more fruit and try new varieties. Eat it raw or cook it; forget canned fruit.
- Use artificial sweeteners, but use caution as some have adverse side effects.
- Eat foods in their natural state without sauce, salt, or sugar. Most foods lose flavor when they are drowned in these additions.
- Start buying yourself treats of food that are not sweet. These can be any food that you love that you never buy because it is expensive or because it never occurs to you. Try an avocado, some imported cheese, or a gourmet take-out soup. Get a small amount and savor it.
- Drink juices and water instead of soda. Beware of diet sodas, as most are loaded with salt and chemicals. Try a salt-free sparkling mineral water.
- Buy unsweetened cereals. Use yogurt instead of ice cream. Try plain yogurt or half-plain and half-flavored.
- When you eat meat, you may get a craving for something sweet. So you may want to cut down on meat.

17

When you greatly reduce your intake of sugar, you change your tolerance level for it. Foods that are slightly sweet taste very sweet, and foods that are very sweet become sickening.

(b) Carbohydrates

Replace all white bread with whole grain bread, such as rye, whole wheat, oatmeal, and corn. These are high in fiber, which means they are more filling and provide nourishment without added fat. They also have more flavor than white bread. Be sure to read labels if you buy commercial brands, as many are high in salt. Some are only partly whole grain and have a deceptive label.

For the same reasons, replace all white rice and white pasta with brown rice and whole grain products which contain complex carbohydrates. Complex carbohydrates are high in fiber and provide a large amount of protein. This includes all beans; whole wheat, artichoke, and corn pastas; chick peas; barley; and bulgar wheat.

Add herbs or tomato sauce to these grain products for added flavor, and buy vegetarian cookbooks for recipes. Try some of these items as between meal snacks, too.

(c) Chocolate

Because chocolate is chemically addictive and is very high in fat, you need to give it up. You can easily replace it with carob.

Carob comes from a tree, and it is low in fat. It is sold as a powder to use in milkshakes, candy bars, pudding, and ice cream. The taste is similar to chocolate, except it is more bitter. It will not, however, taste like chocolate while you still eat chocolate. But once you have given up chocolate, you'll find carob a satisfactory substitute.

Because it is bitter, carob products are sold with a lot of sugar or honey to sweeten them. You must read labels or ask for unsweetened candy bars. Of course, if you eat the whole bar instead of a portion of it, you will have consumed a lot of calories. But there is no chemical addiction and no blood sugar havoc if the carob is unsweetened.

(d) Salt

Salt causes fluid retention and plays a role in hypertension. You will feel and look better if you lower your salt intake. When you do, you will lower your tolerance level for salt, and foods with salt in them will seem too salty.

To lower your salt intake, try the following:
- Use herbs to flavor food.
- Read labels for all processed foods, which generally have a high level of salt.

- Buy unsalted crackers and low-salt cheese.
- Never add table salt to what you eat.
- Stay away from diet sodas that have a high sodium content.

Chart #1 summarizes these suggestions for you.

CHART #1
FOOD SUBSTITUTION

MEAL	EAT:	INSTEAD OF:
BREAKFAST	-Granola, oatmeal -Egg with whole grain bread -Herb tea, decaffeinated coffee	-Sugar cereals -White bread -Coffee, tea
LUNCH	-Whole grain bread -Turkey, tuna -Salad -Fresh fruit -Unsweetened yogurt	-White bread -Packaged meats -Pasta, pizza -Canned fruit -Sweet yogurt, ice cream, cake
DINNER	-Brown rice, beans, lentils, chick peas, barley -Baked potato -Chicken, fish	-White rice, pasta -French fries -Fatty red meat
OTHER	-Soy margarine -Fruit juice, water -Unsweetened carob -Plain popcorn	-Butter -Soda -Chocolate -Candy, cake

4. Choosing foods that satisfy

You may have decided to replace some of the foods you now eat with healthier ones. But what if you do not always know what you like, or you think you like everything? What if you have never been discriminating before?

Chances are that what you do with food is what you do in most areas of your life: you act without examining if that act is right for you or your needs, be it choosing clothes, decorating your home, choosing a career, or maybe even friends or a mate. So why would you give that much thought to what you eat?

When you make more choices in other areas of your life, you will become more choosy about food. (How to deal with your

19

emotional needs is discussed in chapter 5.) It is also true that when you think more before you reach for a food about whether it is exactly the one you want, you will soon begin to realize what you feel about other areas of your life.

The next time you shop for food —

(a) Make a list of exactly what you want to get, so you won't be tempted to buy on impulse.

(b) Buy only the brands you like best, even if it means going to more than one market. YOU DESERVE IT!

(c) Read labels carefully to see what you are going to put into your body.

(d) Buy small amounts. Next time you may want something different.

When you are hungry and go to the refrigerator or to a restaurant, you should choose foods that are exactly what you want at that moment. You should not settle for less. You should not choose according to a prescribed list, nor should you plan meals a week or even days in advance.

Keep a variety of foods in the house, or shop frequently. When you are not sure what you want, close your eyes and try to get in touch with the KIND of food you want. Ask yourself these questions:

- Do I want something HOT or COLD (temperature)?
- Do I want something LIQUID or SOLID (consistency)?
- Do I want something SWEET, SALTY, BITTER, or SOUR (taste)?
- Do I want something SMOOTH and creamy or HARD and chewy (texture)?

It doesn't matter what the food is, as long as it fits the description. If you eat when you are thirsty, or settle for ice cream when you want a chewy food, you will eat more because you remain unsatisfied.

Try eating exactly the kinds of foods you want at every meal for a week, and see if, as a result, you eat less.

c. WHEN YOU EAT

Most people don't overeat at every meal or every time they snack. For example, you might eat three sensible meals a day, but perhaps you binge on a bedtime snack every night. If you can discover *when* you overeat, you can begin to understand why and be on the road to stopping it.

Look at the following examples of common times for people to overeat.

1. At various times during the day

• *When the clock says it's time to eat:* Do you look at the clock and then reach for food when you see noon or 1 p.m., and again at 5 or 6 p.m.? If so, you are responding automatically to an external signal rather than to an internal one. This is an adult version of scheduled feeding done in infancy.

The problem with eating by the clock is that you learn to ignore your inner clock, and if you get hungry at the "wrong" time, you feel guilty. Other times you will eat at the "right" time when you are not yet hungry. Soon you turn off all your inner signals, as they just confuse you.

Eating by the clock continues long after infancy. As a child, you were told in school when to have lunch, and chances are your dinner was at a set time. When you went to work, you were given a set lunch hour. All this is part of our civilized lifestyle, but it makes eating an automatic action, rather than a choice based on hunger.

You eat by the clock because you were taught to do so, but also because it may be more convenient or because it fits into your schedule. You also do it because you get lazy. You avoid having to make a decision about eating. Once you give up your decision-making power, you risk overeating.

• *Late at night:* If you are on the go all day and then come home and collapse, or keep going until after dinner and then collapse, you may find that being tired triggers you to reach for food. There is nothing mysterious about why this happens. When you are tired, your body seeks renewed energy. Often, food can give it to you, but only if you have not eaten in a long time. It would be better to rest first. That is more likely what your body wants.

But, you ask, how can I rest when I have so much to do? You can and must, even if it is only for 10 minutes. It will give you renewed energy, and you will accomplish much more than if you didn't do it.

Instead of being tired, you may be all keyed up late at night and need to unwind. When you take in food, your system slows down to focus on digesting the food. Then you feel less keyed up, and the next time you are tense you associate it with a need to eat. Of course, then you get fat and feel guilty about the eating.

There are alternatives to this pattern:

(a) Make yourself sit down in a comfortable chair, close your eyes for about 20 minutes, breathe deeply and *meditate* or *daydream*. Let the thoughts flow without censoring them.

(b) Put on your sneakers and run or walk around the block; take the dog out; do sit-ups on the floor.

(c) Put on a dumb TV program and stare at it for half an hour, but don't have any food with you.

21

(d) Take a nap. If this makes you feel guilty, set the alarm to limit it. If it is possible, just go to sleep for the night.

The most important thing is to recognize what your body is saying. If it is saying you are tired, the appropriate response is REST, not food.

Some people eat late at night because it is their only opportunity to sit down without the interruptions of children, chores, or the telephone. If this is your pattern, you may need to change some daily routines:

(a) Make this night meal your dinner. Don't eat earlier when things are hectic, or only eat part of the meal then.

(b) If you have a baby, eat only when the baby is napping.

(c) Get in the habit of taking the phone off the hook any time you eat.

(d) Give eating importance, and do not allow others to interrupt you when you eat. Tell your children, "I'm eating now. You'll have to wait."

• *When you are alone:* When eating becomes secretive, it becomes more exciting and more difficult to give up. If you allow those you live with to monitor what you eat and make comments about it, it is time to become more assertive. It is not the business of another person to tell you anything about your eating. It is up to you to say that. If you do, others will soon know to leave you alone.

It may be that no one makes any comments to you or even cares what you do. It may be that when you were a child someone did. Perhaps your parents thought you were fat and measured what you could have or gave you nasty looks if you wanted a second helping. Maybe you even live alone now and there is no one to see you eat, but as a child you got in the habit of being a sneak eater. You ate late at night when no one was around to see you. If you do that now it is from habit and not necessity.

The act of eating is not a sin. Even eating too much isn't. It may be out of habit or because of emotional needs. The first step to overcoming overeating is to go public with it, so it loses the furtive quality.

• *When you are over-hungry:* It may be that when you come home from work, not only are you tired, but you are really very hungry. If you did not eat much all day because you were too busy, or because you like to show others that you are dieting, by the evening you will be starved. If you are, you will eat a lot, and gain more than if you spaced out the same amount of food over a day. Your body cannot burn as much when you sleep.

If you work, it would be better to eat a large lunch, for that is the time when you are most active. If you have a sedentary job, this might not be the best idea, and you should eat moderately all day.

In any case, do not create a situation where you are overly hungry because you did not eat enough during the day.

• *When you are bored:* Do you eat because you are bored and have nothing better to do? It may be that you have too much free time and feel angry about it. You may have feelings about other things in your life that you don't want to face, and when you turn off your feelings, you do become bored. If you eat out of boredom, find other activities to do with your extra time, especially creative ones that you enjoy.

• *When you are lonely:* If you feel too alone and then deal with it by reaching for food, you do not end up being less lonely. You need to bring people into your life. You may eat because of the memories you have about people and food from childhood. Try daydreaming about those times without eating now.

• *When you want to avoid chores:* You may find that you eat every time you have to do something you would like to avoid, such as laundry, housecleaning, or homework. You allow yourself to postpone the task when you sit down to eat. Why not just allow yourself a break before doing the chore; sit down without eating? If you are like many other people, you feel more guilty about "wasting" the time by relaxing than by eating when you aren't hungry.

• *When you watch television:* Eating while you watch TV is a habit reinforced by food commercials. It helps to have the TV far from the kitchen, or make a rule for yourself that you will only eat at the table in the kitchen area.

• *When you read:* You tend to eat more when you are not aware you are eating. Both reading and watching television divert your attention away from whether you are full. Also, when you read, you don't really tune in to the taste of your food and you have to eat more to feel satisfied. Sometimes eating is an excuse to sit and read when you feel guilty about taking the time to read. You tell yourself that it is all right to take time to eat, when all you really want to do is read.

• *When others eat:* It may be that you eat moderately except when food is in front of you. When you see someone in your family eating, you eat too. Some of that is the result of being with people who want others to eat with them the way some people want others to drink with them. Or it may be that you feel left out unless you eat too, as eating has become a social experience. There is no reason, however, why you cannot sit at a table with anyone and share in the conversation without eating. Does that seem rude to you? If so, just explain why you are doing it. If, for instance, you don't eat dinner until your spouse comes home, but by that time you have nibbled out of hunger, just say that to eat again would mean a weight gain for you.

So when is eating appropriate? The only time to eat is WHEN YOU ARE HUNGRY. (See chapter 4 on hunger.)

For one week keep track of when you reach for food. Use Exercise #4 to see what your pattern is.

EXERCISE #4
WHEN YOU EAT

For each day, write down every time you eat anything, what the situation was at the time (e.g., watching TV, feeling lonely), and what you ate.

DAY	TIME OF DAY	SITUATION OR HOW YOU FELT	WHAT YOU ATE
Monday			
Tuesday			
Wednesday			
Thursday			
Friday			
Saturday			
Sunday	1130-1200	while studying	2 cream cheese sandwiches 1 apple

2. At meals

If you have discovered that most of your eating is done at times other than mealtime, you need to look at what happens when you're eating meals. The more enjoyment you get from meals, the less you will tend to eat in between them.

24

What is your favorite meal? What is your least favorite? Do you know why? Here are some possible reasons you may have for liking or disliking a meal.

(a) Breakfast
- You can eat it without guilt because you have not eaten yet that day.
- You can really enjoy it because you are hungry.
- You enjoy being able to eat it alone.

If breakfast is not your favorite meal, it may be because you eat too much at bedtime so you are never hungry for breakfast; or you have to rush through it, as you must get ready for work. It may be a meal you skip. Maybe you do not like the choices of breakfast foods. Or maybe you feel too pressured in the morning to eat with your family who expect you to fix their breakfast, and each one wants something different at a different time.

To get more pleasure out of breakfast, try to —
- Find new foods to include. Elsewhere in the world people eat potatoes, tomatoes, cheeses, and meats at breakfast.
- Make an effort to eat less at night so you can feel hungry for breakfast.
- Get up earlier to have more time to enjoy it.
- Wait to eat breakfast until the family has left the house.

(b) Lunch
- You enjoy not having to cook anything.
- You can eat it with friends at work. You like going out.
- You get to eat it alone; you enjoy reading while you eat.
- You like the choices of foods for lunch.

If lunch is not a pleasure to you, it may be because you only let yourself have a salad and are bored with it; maybe you hate eating alone; maybe you feel self-conscious when you go out to eat with co-workers because you think they are watching what you eat.

To get more pleasure out of lunch, try to —
- Find new foods to eat without feeling guilty about them.
- Invite a friend to lunch.
- Remember that no one is interested in your eating; they are most likely on a diet and self-conscious too.

(c) Dinner
- You like the foods available.
- You like to cook.
- You like having the whole family eating together.

- You feel really hungry after starving yourself all day.
- You get a chance to talk to your spouse.

If dinner is your least favorite meal, maybe it is because you hate to cook, or you dislike the foods you allow yourself to eat and see the rest of the family eat those you love. Maybe the family fights at the table so dinner is a tense meal. Maybe they seem to resent the time spent together or are in a hurry. Maybe you feel too full at dinner because of snacking all day.

To get more pleasure out of dinner, try to —

- Find simple recipes, especially casseroles.
- Make the foods you love in a less fattening way, e.g., substitute skim milk for cream in a recipe.
- Have the family eat together, but allow members to leave the table as soon as they finish the meal.
- Never cook separate meals for anyone or serve more than once a night. If your spouse gets home late, either wait to eat or have part of the meal earlier.
- If you do not enjoy eating alone every night, invite a friend to dinner, read, or set the table as though you were a guest.

d. WHERE YOU EAT

Where do you eat? To eat less, you need to confine all your eating to one place only: AT THE TABLE (kitchen or dining room) and only while sitting down. You will eat less because you will be more aware that you are eating.

Pay attention to all the places where you now eat. Look at the following examples of common locations where people eat. Where do you eat?

- *At the stove:* You tell yourself you have to taste what you are cooking, and so you sample a little. But then you repeat the taste every few minutes. By the time you serve dinner, you are full, but you eat again. You may do this because as a child your mother let you sample her cooking and doing so now with your own evokes memories. Or, you may enjoy eating out of the pot more than eating at the table with your family because you feel self-conscious when you eat with them. Perhaps you eat too little lunch and are too hungry when you cook. Try eating a larger lunch, or let the food you have eaten from the pot count as a meal and don't eat dinner.
- *In front of TV:* Eating in front of the TV is usually a habit that began when you were a child. As stated before, be sure the TV is far from the kitchen. If you must snack, go to the kitchen during a commercial and eat there.

- *In the bedroom:* There are several reasons why you may eat in the bedroom:
  - (a) As an infant you were fed in the bedroom in your mother's arms or in your crib. When you eat in bed now you are symbolically reverting to infancy and a time of comfort.
  - (b) The bedroom is where sex and intimacy take place, so you are using food as a substitute sensual experience when you are lonely.
  - (c) Your room is a place where you can eat in secret, in privacy. It may be that you have no other activity in your life that you feel is just yours, so you need to do something special. It could be reading, painting, or anything that is pleasurable, but you have chosen eating.

- *In the car:* Eating in the car can stem from childhood when you were given a cookie on a family outing to keep you quiet. It became a habit that needs to be broken.

e. WHY YOU EAT

You are overeating if you eat when you are not hungry. Some of the reasons you might do this stem from the way food was handled in your childhood. These old messages and patterns need to be recognized so that you can consciously reject them and change your attitude toward eating.

Which of the following childhood situations apply to you? Think about how they have affected your current eating patterns.

- (a) Every time you cried, you were given a cookie, which you now interpret to mean that *food can comfort you* and that *it is not good to feel unhappy.*
- (b) Perhaps you were ignored when you cried to be fed. Your mother may have been too busy or believed that crying was good for you. You soon learned that being hungry was frightening. As a result, you may now eat constantly to avoid re-experiencing hunger.
- (c) Your mother gave you a lot of food, and she acted hurt if you turned it down. When you are offered food by anyone, you never say no, as you expect they will feel hurt if you do.
- (d) Your parents praised restraint, which you now interpret to mean that *acting on impulse shows weakness.* So when you binge, you feel like a failure.
- (e) You were expected to clean your plate, which you now interpret to mean that *wasting food is a sin.* So you always eat everything that is there.

(f) No one in your family expressed anger. Instead, they ate to push away such feelings. So when you feel angry now, you eat.

(g) Eating was always done at set times, so now you eat by the clock. The implication is that it is wrong, even dangerous, to be spontaneous.

(h) Whenever you were "good," you received a treat of candy, cake, or some sweet. You now associate sweets with being good.

(i) Everyone ate quickly because eating was not viewed as very important. Now eating fast is a habit for you.

(j) Eating was considered a very important activity, and much time was spent doing it. You find it hard now not to make it a high priority.

The patterns developed in childhood affect the way you think about food now. And the way you think about food affects how much you eat. You can replace the old messages you received about food with new, more appropriate ones. Look at Exercise #5 and check off which old messages you believe. Then read what the truth is about them and begin to tell yourself the new messages.

EXERCISE #5
MESSAGES ABOUT FOOD AND EATING

OLD MESSAGE	TRUTH	NEW MESSAGE
☐Food will make me fat.	Excess food makes you fat, giving you calories that you don't burn. You can lose weight by eating any food, even ice cream, if your total calorie consumption is low.	Too much food will make me fat.
☐Foods are good or bad.	Foods have no moral value. You are not good or bad for what you eat. Some foods are better or worse for your health.	Foods can be good or bad *for me*.
☐If I eat little, I am good.	How much you eat depends on paying attention to your stomach. If you ignore your hunger and do not eat, you are not better than someone who responds to hunger by eating. Nor are you bad if you overeat. You are using food to cope with life.	How much I eat has nothing to do with my worth.
☐Overeating means I am out of control.	Eating when you are full shows too much control, not letting your stomach dictate to you. You need to listen to your body.	Overeating shows me I have to learn new ways to cope.
☐My appearance tells me how much to eat.	Eating too much or too little affects your health, so you must listen to your body.	If I am healthy from eating the amount my stomach truly needs, I will look great.
☐Food can make me feel better.	Not if you hate yourself for eating it.	I can make myself feel better by praising myself.
☐Eating is the only activity I have a right to take time out for.	It is O.K. to do nothing at times. You will actually do better at work if you take time to play. Eating is not a good substitute for play.	I have a right to take time out any way I wish.

4

UNDERSTANDING HUNGER

When your stomach is empty, it requires food to give you energy, and signals are sent to your brain. You may have a gnawing, growling, or acid feeling. You may feel shaky or faint. You may feel pain.

How frequently these sensations occur depends on many factors: how much you recently ate, how fast you burned it up, how active you were. Usually hunger occurs several hours after a meal.

Do Exercise #6 to pinpoint the kind of hunger you experience.

EXERCISE #6
HUNGER PROFILE

1. When I am hungry, the sensations I have are:

    ____ gnawing   ✓ acid   ____ headache

    ____ dizziness   ✓ fatigue   ✓ emptiness

2. I know when I am hungry:

    ____ always   ____ never   ✓ most of the time

3. When I feel hungry, I:

    ✓ am scared   ____ am pleased

    ____ must eat   ____ can wait

a. CAUSES OF HUNGER

An empty stomach is only one cause of hunger. Another may be food itself. For example, if you have an allergic reaction to certain food, eating that food may make you feel hungry. If you have low blood sugar, eating something high in carbohydrates will make you hungry. A breakfast of muffins, toast, bagels or most sweet cereals will trigger hunger faster than eggs, meat or cheese. Combining some fat with a protein food will slow down digestion and keep you less hungry.

For women, feeling hungry just before your menstrual period is normal. It is important for compulsive eaters to know this and to check the calendar. Try to eat more protein rather than carbo-hydrates at such times. If you get the blues and crave sugar to make you feel better, try instead to eat foods that will raise your estrogen level: eggs, milk products, and legumes.

b. REACTING TO HUNGER

When you feel hungry, how do you react? Are you delighted to think you most likely did not overeat earlier? Do you consider the hunger a natural part of being alive? Do you let yourself feel the hunger, or do you run to eat? What if you are in the middle of doing something? Do you feel panic? Are you afraid you will pass out? How long do you think you could go without eating before you got a headache or before you passed out? For some it is 24 hours. If you feel really sick after just two or three hours, you may be hypoglycemic, that is, have low blood sugar.

Do you ever feel hungry and purposely ignore it? Are you just too busy to eat, or do you actually think you are a stronger person for having done so? Or do you eat by the clock, and so decide that your stomach must be wrong?

Digestion is an involuntary process. If you are hungry in the middle of the morning or in the late afternoon, consider one of the previous causes. You might want to check your diet, your metabolism, or your blood sugar. Consistently ignoring hunger is foolish; your body is trying to tell you something, and you should listen to the message.

c. FEELING FULL AND NOT EATING

Hunger tells you when to start eating. Feeling full tells you when to stop. It is natural to stop eating when hunger is gone. But do you know when that is?

If you eat very fast, there is no time for your stomach to send signals to your brain to stop eating. If you do other activities while eating, such as talking on the phone or reading, you cannot pay attention to how your stomach feels. If you eat by the clock, you may be eating at times when you are not hungry.

No matter how frequently you eat, or how much you eat at one time, there is some point at which you stop. When is that? Is it when you are so full that it hurts? Is it when all the food is gone from your plate? Is it when an item of food is gone from your home? Is it when you are mildly uncomfortable? If you can pin-point your stopping point, you can begin to change it. If you stop eating at any time other than when hunger is gone, you are eating in an unnatural way that may be unhealthy.

d. SHARPENING YOUR AWARENESS

You may never actually feel hungry, especially if you eat frequently. You may have completely lost touch with the signals from your stomach. To increase your hunger awareness, try these suggestions:

(a) Several times a day, close your eyes and focus on how your stomach feels. Are you hungry? How do you know?

(b) Wait a while before eating, especially breakfast, so you can experience your hunger. Instead of eating the moment you get up, wait half an hour. Get dressed, do the things you usually do after eating. Pay attention to how your stomach feels. See if your hunger increases. Eat more for breakfast and lunch. See if you are less hungry for dinner. Eat nothing after dinner. You should wake up hungry.

(c) Eat half of a meal, then get up from the table and walk around the room for a few minutes. See if you are still hungry and still want to eat more.

(d) Skip a meal if you are not hungry. But do eat if you are hungry. That is better than waiting until the evening to eat, ignoring your hunger during the day. You will get too hungry and will eat more than your body can efficiently burn in one sitting.

(e) Eat slowly so that your brain can communicate with your stomach. If necessary, use gimmicks to slow yourself down:
  - Eat with the other hand.
  - Use chopsticks.
  - Put down the fork between bites.
  - Eat with a mirror on the table in front of you.

(f) Put smaller portions on your plate. Before taking more, think about how your stomach feels.

(g) Any time you reach for food, ask yourself, "Am I really hungry?"

e. EMOTIONAL HUNGER

How can you tell if what you are feeling is the result of an empty stomach or an empty life? Consider when you last ate. If it was recently and you feel hungry, you may want something other than food. Or you may be reaching for food to avoid doing something you dread. Ask yourself what alternatives you have to eating.

When you have an emotional need, you want something. You have a void you want to fill. You want to be fulfilled. Instead, you fill yourself with food. You believe your life is full when your stomach is. You have become addicted to that full feeling in your stomach, and to the concept of feeling full.

Some people associate hunger with poverty: a full stomach means a full wallet. Hunger can mean being needy or dependent.

When you realize that you reach for food because of something you are feeling emotionally rather than physically, that awareness can help you change. The goal is to substitute new ways to deal with your feelings instead of using food. Until you can do that, it is helpful to understand which foods are the most appropriate for which feeling and most directly satisfy the need the feelings imply. (See Chart #2.)

CHART #2
FOODS TO FILL NEEDS

FEELING	NEED	SATISFYING FOODS	REASONS
Lonely	Nurturing	Smooth foods (ice cream, butter, peanut butter) Warm foods (soup, tea, milk)	Suggest infancy Suggest warmth
Deprived	Pleasure	Sweets	Give pleasure
Bored	Excitement	Spicy foods	Add zest
Angry	Release	Hard, chewy foods (carrot, meat, breadstick)	Involve the teeth
Tired	Energy	Carbohydrates, sweets	Raise blood sugar
Sexual	Sensual experience	Sweets (chocolate, any food you like)	Satisfy senses
Unloved	Strokes	Sweets (any food you love)	Suggest reward, treat

If you identify your need, and then pick a food that directly satisfies that need, you are likely to eat less. (Remember also to eat slowly in order to derive the most benefit from any food you choose.)

Of course, your satisfaction can only be temporary when you use food to feed the emotions. Your ultimate goal is to deal with your emotions in ways other than through food.

33

5

EMOTIONS AND EATING HABITS

Your emotions, or feelings, can be mild, vague, intense, pleasant, or unpleasant. You have many feelings: anger, unhappiness, fear, joy, happiness, confusion, anxiety. These feelings are neither good nor bad; you cannot attach a moral value to your feelings. Simply, your feelings are what make you human.

However, it is not uncommon for people to try to stop feeling because they have been taught that it is good to avoid unpleasant feelings or that if they do not rid themselves of negative feelings, they will be destroyed. One common way to try to push aside feelings is by eating.

When you try to escape from what you are feeling, that feeling generally grows larger. You develop physical symptoms, such as pain in your throat, upset stomach, headache, insomnia, or depression. Repressing your feelings causes your body more strain than coping with them. Crying or yelling, for example, are ways to release the tension you feel. When you are scared and admit it, you feel less scared. When you vent your anger, it is gone.

Sometimes, you cannot remedy an upsetting situation immediately, and you need a temporary aid. Instead of using food, try some of these positive ways to deal with your immediate feelings:

- Exercise
- Read
- Meditate
- Watch TV
- Cry
- Shop
- Write poetry or in a journal
- Daydream
- Paint
- Take a bath
- Take a walk
- Call a friend

The next time you reach for food to deal with a problem, stop yourself and use one of these methods instead. To prepare for doing that, do Exercise #7. Then use the information in the following sections to learn to deal directly with your emotions.

EXERCISE #7
FEELINGS AND FOOD CHECKLIST

Look at the list of emotions. Write down what food, if any, you turn to in reaction to these emotions. Then write down a new way to deal with the feeling.		
When I feel:	The food I eat is:	Instead of eating I could do the following:
Lonely		
Afraid		
Angry		
Bored		
Frustrated		
In conflict		
Rejected		
Depressed		

a. ANXIETY

Anxiety is a vague state of unrest and apprehension. When you feel anxious, ask yourself, "What am I upset about? What is the feeling?" When you have identified the feeling, you need to know:

(a) Is there some action you can take to remedy this situation?

(b) Is the situation causing this distress beyond your control? If so, you must learn to accept it.

(c) Is the situation temporary? Almost every situation is, especially if it is a crisis. If it is, it will pass. We usually recover from illness, from mourning a loss, from what we fear. Bad situations improve. LIFE IS CHANGE.

You do not need to panic about a situation. Allow yourself to feel the anxiety, knowing that it will pass. You do not need to reach for food. If you must escape for the moment, use one of the positive methods suggested above.

Situations and feelings do pass. The only time feelings do not change is when a person is "clinically depressed." In that case, professional counseling is needed.

b. ANGER

What made you angry as a child? Was it being constantly criticized by a parent? Were you then angry with the other parent for not putting a stop to it? Were you angry with a sibling for teasing you or for getting more attention or love than you? Were you angry about being told what to do? Think about your past and present reactions to anger and fill in Exercise #8.

EXERCISE #8
ANGER QUESTIONNAIRE

1. As a child, I became angry when: _being criticized_
   being left alone

2. When I was angry I would:
   ____have a temper tantrum   ____hit someone
   _✓_run away   ____be insolent
   _✓_sulk or cry   ____rebel

3. When I expressed my anger I was:
   _✓_ignored   ____rejected
   ____punished   ____listened to

4. Now I become angry when: _others assume for me_
   and I let them.

5. When I am angry, I:
   ____yell and scream   _✓_overeat
   _✓_cry   ____confront the issue
   ____become sarcastic

6. As a result, I usually:
   ____hurt someone   ____feel relieved
   _✓_feel hurt   _✓_feel out of control
   ____get rejected   ____am ignored

7. I wish instead that when I get angry I would: _confront the_
   issue

36

Knowing how you deal with anger is the first step to being able to change it if you want.

1. Expressing anger

What did you do about the anger you felt as a child? Did you feel it was safe to express this anger? Your mother may have taken such anger as a rejection of her. So she let you know that she did not want it, that you were not to verbalize it. Perhaps she never showed her anger. So you thought the anger you felt meant you had a problem.

In any case, if you buried your anger as a child, you learned to lose touch with your feelings. After a while, you may have stopped even realizing you were angry.

Do you still repress your anger as an adult? Are you being taken for granted by family members? Is your boss too demanding? Are others invading your privacy? Are you feeling angry about the same kind of things that angered you as a child?

If you do not express your anger, you probably base that repression on a lot of misconceptions:

- *My anger will destroy the other person.* If you think this, you think you are very powerful. Actually, the only thing your anger can do is upset someone or make them angry. Expressing feelings openly leads eventually to a better relationship. Perhaps you really think you are the one who will be destroyed if your anger is met with anger. But you, as well as others, are stronger than you think.

- *If I express anger, I will lose control and look like a fool.* This only happens when you store the anger up too long. If you express your anger rationally and calmly when you feel it, you will not lose control.

- *If I express anger, I will be rejected.* People who feel threatened by your anger may reject you in defense. This means that they have a problem, not that you did something wrong. If you hide your anger, people may feel safer with you, but this does not guarantee their love.

- *I have no right to express anger to a good person.* A good person deserves your honesty, not pretense.

- *No one will listen to me unless I yell.* When you yell, people are more likely to tune you out. Perhaps, as a child, you got your way by having temper tantrums. That is no longer necessary. You can simply say how you feel.

- *If I ignore my anger, it will go away. I can divert it with food.* Unexpressed feelings stay with you. If you overeat, you turn the anger against yourself. It is still there.

Repressed anger causes depression and illness. There is a build-up of energy that needs release. This is when anger can turn to rage. Try Exercise #9 to help you understand how you react to anger.

EXERCISE #9
ANGER FANTASY

Make yourself comfortable. Be sure that you will not be interrupted. Close your eyes and visualize someone who has made you angry in the past or someone you still feel angry at. See that person sitting in a chair near you. Tell that person all you feel about him or her. Let it all out. Use physical force if you wish.

Be aware of how your body feels when you release this anger. After the fantasy, consider what you said, and how you felt. Did you use force? If not, did you want to? Would you ever really push someone? Why did you not say these things to this person in real life?

2. Anger and eating

Feeling angry will cause you to eat only if you do not express that anger. Food kills some of the anger energy you feel. It momentarily makes you too full to move or to feel. It fills the void left by the unfinished business of the angry feelings. Until you deal directly with your anger, you feel unsatisfied. This dissatisfaction is a kind of "hunger."

If you do not tell the person you are angry at how you feel, he or she is not likely to treat you any differently next time. You have to change your response to that person before there will be any change. Instead of eating when you are angry, say the following things to yourself.

- I have a right to get angry.
- I can express my anger without losing control.
- I can tell someone I am angry and not be hurtful.
- I can be heard when I express my anger.
- I can get angry and still be loved.
- If I express my anger, I will eat less.

3. Becoming detached

When you think everyone else's behavior is caused by you or directed to you in some way, you take things too personally and overreact. Then you are constantly angry. You need to be more objective about other people's motives. You need to change some of your expectations about the world.

(a) Stop expecting the world to be fair. There is much injustice in our society; many people are selfish; many are manipulators. You need to see clearly who is actually trying to hurt you and act to stop it without attempting to reform the whole world, and without expecting to be treated fairly by everyone.

(b) Stop thinking the world owes you something. Life is what you make it. Others are not on this earth to cater to you. If you give love, you will most likely get love. If you walk around angry, with a chip on your shoulder, you will not receive love.

(c) Stop thinking you have been chosen for unfair treatment. While a few people may at times be angry with you or out to get you, most people are not even aware of your existence.

(d) Start wondering what has really caused the other person's behavior. Perhaps he is scolding you because he is upset about his child's illness and just is in a rotten mood. Perhaps you remind her of her sister who irritated her when she was a child. It may not be you that the other person is reacting to specifically.

(e) Decide if it is appropriate to express anger. If telling your boss you are angry jeopardizes your job, you may want to hold it in. If your father has a heart condition, upsetting him may not be smart. If your sister is leaving the country next week, this may not be the time to confront her. On the other hand, you may want to express your anger to those you care about and have to deal with every day.

(f) Decide if the situation can be changed by expressing your anger. It is useless to get angry about the weather or a traffic jam or the assignment the teacher gave or the washing machine that broke down. Some situations can be changed; perhaps moving, getting divorced, or leaving your job solves the problem. Confrontation of another with your anger may be needed at first, but after a while, action may be more appropriate. If anger consumes you, you cannot take action or be objective or even evaluate the situation.

By changing your thinking, you can become more detached and less angry. This does not mean you need to repress your anger. It means you won't even get angry except when appropriate. And when is it appropriate? When your rights are being denied, you are directly affected, and you know that confrontation can mean change. However, if you follow the guidelines above, you will probably feel angry less often. Less anger to repress or express can mean less eating.

4. Defiant eating

It may be that your eating is in itself an expression of anger, rather than a way to stifle your anger. Perhaps, as a child, you were overweight and food was restricted. Your mother meant well and was concerned about your health, but you did not appreciate her concern. You felt resentful and thought to yourself, "I'll show her." And you did by sneaking food and eating defiantly. You may be still doing it despite her lack of involvement in your eating habits.

Or perhaps your spouse complains about your pot belly and wants you to diet. You eat just because someone wants you to cut down on your eating.

How can you stop eating as an angry act? Consider how you are hurting yourself, since you want to lose weight, and you really want to eat less. Then do the following:

- Keep to yourself information about your weight and your eating.
- Tell the other person how you feel when that person voices an opinion.
- Do only what *you* want to do for you; don't try to please or defy another.

EXPRESS YOUR ANGER WITH WORDS, NOT FOOD.

c. ASSERTIVENESS

The healthy way to express anger is to be assertive. Assertiveness is not aggressiveness, nor is it passivity.

When you are aggressive, you control others and they resent you for it. They must fight you or become your victim. You end up lonely and unhappy. No one loves a bully, not even the bully. When you are aggressive, communication is not possible.

When you are passive, you express your anger by calling yourself names, by turning the anger inward, and by blaming yourself. You protect yourself from dealing with the other person. The other person does not find out what you are feeling, so there can be no changes made. You see yourself as a victim, and the world takes advantage of you.

But when you are assertive, you have an impact on others and they have an impact on you. You have vitality and make your own decisions, but you are aware that others exist. You talk about your feelings and actions. You do not expect others to exist just for you, and you do not expect to exist just for them.

Being assertive means that you believe you are equal to the other person. You convey this with your whole body. You look the other person in the eye. You hold your body erect. You keep your head straight, not down. You speak in a firm voice.

If you feel you have to attack to be heard, you will look threatening, and speak too loudly. Your eyes will bulge, your face will get red, and you will scowl. The other person will not want to deal with you.

Apologizing for your behavior is not being assertive. It implies that you do not think too much of yourself. Why then would anyone else? If you really are not sorry and know you did the right thing, don't apologize just to avoid confronting the other person.

In order to be assertive, you must first know that you have a right to be. You have many rights, some of which you share with all other people. These include the right to privacy, to make mistakes, to get respect, and to have your feelings.

What rights do you have that are special for you? Make a list of them. How many of them do you make sure are honored? People will treat you the way you expect them to, the way you let them know you want.

Complete the assertiveness profile in Exercise #10.

EXERCISE #10
ASSERTIVENESS PROFILE

From the words given, choose the most appropriate one to complete each thought.

(spouse, lover, friend, employer, parent, child, doctor, waiter, clerk)

I am most assertive with _____ _friend_ _____.

I am least assertive with _____ _parent_ _____.

(love, attention, directions, money, job)

I am most assertive when asking for _____ _directions_ _____.

I am least assertive when asking for _____ _love_ _____.

(love, praise, anger, rights)

I am most assertive when expressing _____ _praise_ _____.

I am least assertive when expressing _____ _anger_ _____.

Are you assertive with people who are close to you, such as friends and relatives? Is it easier for you to be assertive with people you don't know well? Do you feel that people you know are more predictable, that you know how they will react, so it is safer to be assertive with them?

Do you find it easy or difficult to ask for something impersonal, such as directions? Is it even harder for you to ask for personal things, such as love, sex, or attention?

The people in your life cannot know what you want unless you tell them. If you ask clearly, they are not likely to turn you down. If you do not get what you want because you don't ask for it, you have no right to be angry with others. They cannot read your mind. They may even think you don't care whether or not they pay attention to you.

Of course, you will not always get what you want, but by asking, you have taken some control over your life.

Can you express your negative feelings? Can you express your positive feelings by giving praise? Perhaps you never thought this was being assertive. Being assertive means being in charge, not being a victim. This can only happen if you are open about all your feelings and all your needs.

d. STRESS

Overeating is one way of coping with stress. You feel upset about something, so you eat to comfort yourself. Eating can make you feel better temporarily. If you could feel upset less often, you could eat less.

Unfortunately, most of the things that are upsetting will not go away. They come from three sources and mostly cannot be eliminated by eating. The three sources are —

(a) *People*, including your family, friends, neighbors, boss, colleagues, teachers, doctors, clerks, mechanics, or restaurant help. They are all part of your life and, no matter what you do, they will continue to be there. The stress comes when they perform inefficiently, or try to control you, or do something that worries you.

(b) *Situations*, including pressures from your job; changes such as the birth of a child, a new job, a marriage, a divorce, a move; financial problems; loss through death; deadlines; conflict; interruption. You might be able to change some of them by leaving your job or changing your schedule. Most of the others you have to live with and deal with as they happen.

(c) *Environment*, including traffic, noise, pollution, crowds, and weather. This only changes if you move or take a vacation.

All these sources of stress, or "stressors," are external. You may aggravate the seriousness of these stressors by how you react internally. This is especially true if your thoughts are distorted, exaggerated, or based on false expectations. If you think, for example, "It's not fair," or "How dare he," or "The world is against me," you will feel rejection, disappointment, anger, guilt, worry, envy, inadequacy, or despair. These negative feelings can lead to eating in an attempt to feel better.

If you can change the way you think about your life, you can begin to feel less stress. You can then also become more willing to make some changes to improve the situations that may be contributing to your stress.

Start by thinking:
- It will pass.
- No one is perfect or needs to be.
- I am responsible for how I react to people and things.
- I can wait to see if it will get better (it usually does).
- Life is not always fair.

You need to accept those situations you cannot change, such as the weather and traffic. And you need to change the situations you cannot accept and are possible to change by, for example, moving to a smaller town, changing your job, or getting a divorce.

In order to have less stress, you need to first know what things upset you. Then you need to know what messages you give yourself about the stressors so you can change those thoughts. It is also important to see if you use food to cope with stressors. Fill out the stress profile in Exercise #11 on page 44 before reading further.

You can now begin to change the way you react to the stressors in your life. Did you identify eating as a means of coping with stress? Understand that one thing you have total control over is what goes into your body. If you eliminate foods that add stress, you will be calmer and better able to deal with the external stressors that come along.

Sugar, caffeine, narcotics, nicotine, additives, alcohol, and allergens (foods you are allergic to) all act as toxins in your body. They can cause depression, restlessness, fatigue, and nervousness. Gentle foods, that is, foods that are easier to digest than heavy, greasy foods, have a calming effect.

Eat foods that are natural, lightly cooked, and very fresh.

EXERCISE #11
STRESS PROFILE

The following external stressors upset me (list several specific ones):	I react with (anger, fear, envy, depression, panic, etc.):	The action I take is to (withdraw, confront, get sick, eat, sleep, etc.):
People (spouse, child, in-law, boss, friend, doctor, clerk, waiter, etc.)		
Jacques Marquis	anger	confront
father	anger depression	withdraw
mother	depression	sleep withdraw
sister	anger	withdraw
Frank	anger	confront
Alicia + Sylvie		confront
Jean-Paul	anger	got sick
Lucien	anger	withdraw
Situations (job, money, sex, change, conflict, criticism, deadlines, noise, etc.)		
job	lack of motivation	ignore
no sex	frustration envy	sleep eat
father's illness	anger/depression/fear	eat sleep

e. DEPRIVATION

Feeling deprived is one of the primary reasons for overeating. Some of these feelings of deprivation come from being deprived as a child — of love, attention, approval. You may still be overeating now as a way to compensate.

As an adult, you may feel deprived of the same things or of things like recognition, friends, wealth. You may give yourself food now because you have not learned how to give yourself anything else. You may believe the following myths:

(a) *I am not entitled to what I want.* As a child, you were probably deprived of love. Instead of feeling anger toward your parents, you told yourself you did not deserve their love. Now, you still tell yourself that about everything you want.

(b) *If I don't take it now, it won't be there later.* As a child, you were probably disappointed many times. So you grew up to believe that waiting was fruitless. Or perhaps you got everything you wanted and never learned to wait. So now, not having instant gratification scares you and overeating reassures you. But the food certainly will be there later, as will most other things you may want now.

(c) *My self-worth is equal to what I have. If I have nothing, I am nothing.* If your self-esteem is low, no matter how much you have, it won't be enough. You will focus on what you don't have and still feel bad about yourself. You will continue to feel deprived and eat to compensate.

The messages you need to have about something you want are: I want it. I deserve it. I will go after it. If it is not available now, I will wait. If it will never be available, I will go after something else.

When you can tell yourself this, you will not need food as a replacement for what you really want.

Give yourself gifts other than food, for example, a nap, phone call, walk, facial, massage, time to read, or anything else you like, but might not do for yourself very often. If you make your life less empty, you will not have to fill it with food. Try doing Exercise #12 for one week and see how it affects your eating.

EXERCISE #12
DAILY GIFTS

Give yourself a gift or reward other than food every day for a week. Record below what you gave yourself and how it affected your eating.

DAY	THE GIFT THAT I GAVE MYSELF:	WHAT EFFECT IT HAD ON MY EATING:
Monday		
Tuesday		
Wednesday		
Thursday		
Friday		
Saturday		
Sunday		

6

TAKING CHARGE OF YOUR LIFE

a. CONTROL

Eating compulsively may make you feel out of control. When you assert yourself, you feel more in control of your life, and you have less need to overeat. When you are in charge of your emotions and stop repressing them you begin to feel better about yourself.

In one sense, you are controlling what and how much you eat even when you are obsessed with food. Society makes food available and then suggests that you eat little and stay thin. If you overeat, you *choose* to ignore these messages. Compulsive eaters *choose* to ignore warnings from doctors about fatty foods, adverse physical reactions to junk foods, diets, and pills.

But if you overeat because someone wants you to be thin, for example, you are controlled by your need to be defiant. You are not eating by choice. You believe that food will solve your problems. Or it may be that you are over-controlled in every area of your life, and eating provides a release from that control. The binge provides a sense of freedom.

Your goal is to take charge of your life and strike a balance between too much control or none at all.

b. BUILDING YOUR SELF-ESTEEM

Do you feel comfortable when someone pays you a compliment? Can you thank them and leave it alone? Or do you —

- add a "but" and negate the compliment? (e.g., "That is a pretty blouse." "But it is so old.")
- tell yourself that if the other person really knew you he or she would not be praising you?
- say something derogatory about yourself that the other person did not notice or might dispute?

Do you ever ask someone what he or she thinks about you, not really wanting to hear anything negative? One way of taking charge of your life is to grow comfortable with both praise and constructive criticism. Fill out the self-esteem profile in Exercise #13 to measure your comfort with self-praise and self-criticism.

EXERCISE #13
SELF-ESTEEM PROFILE

What I like about myself:

1. _____
2. _____
3. _____
4. _____
5. _____
6. _____
7. _____
8. _____
9. _____
10. _____

What I do well:

1. _____
2. _____
3. _____
4. _____
5. _____

What I don't like about myself:

1. _____
2. _____
3. _____
4. _____
5. _____

```
┌─────────────────────────────────────────────────────────┐
│                                                           │
│  What I don't do well:                                    │
│                                                           │
│   1. _____     │
│                                                           │
│   2. _____     │
│                                                           │
│   3. _____     │
│                                                           │
│   4. _____     │
│                                                           │
│   5. _____     │
│                                                           │
└─────────────────────────────────────────────────────────┘
```

Do you find it difficult to praise yourself? Do you feel it is immodest to do so? Actually, it is much more difficult to go through life without first having self-love. When you feel good about who you are, you can face anything: conflict, failure, crisis, decisions. Remember: a diet from living and loving makes a diet from overeating impossible. If you do not love yourself, no one else will; you will feel rejected and you will make up for it with food.

How many good things were you able to write about yourself on the self-esteem profile? Here are some obvious things that you may have overlooked:

• **Intelligence:** Perhaps you don't think you are smart because your knowledge is intuitive rather than factual. If that is so, you can become better informed if you want to. But understand that intuitive knowledge is very valuable, and many well-informed people have not developed their intuition. You need the intuition that tells you what to say to your upset child, what to do in a crisis, how to make a difficult decision. Answers to those issues can't be found in a book. If you are good at these things, you are intelligent. Using your intuition well depends on trusting your feelings.

Also, if you rely on your intuition, you can develop your psychic intelligence. You can pick up cues from your environment: about other people, about your future, about events. You know without knowing how you know. This is an ability that few people use, but anyone can develop. Yours is there, waiting for you to use it.

• **Reliability:** Are you honest? Conscientious? Do you feel bored with those traits, or feel too good? Don't overlook them; not everyone has them. Would you like yourself if you were unreliable? Reliability is a plus. If people lean on you too much because you are so reliable, you simply need to develop your ability to say what your limits are.

- **Sense of humor:** A sense of humor is a wonderful quality, especially if it makes you fun to be around. But if you laugh when you are angry, or unhappy, you are not being true to your feelings, so you probably do not admire this about yourself.

Other qualities you should think about are kindness, curiosity, persistence, and creativity. Are you organized? Are you a good listener? A good parent, spouse, child, or friend? If so, what are the qualities that make you good in these roles? Is it being caring, loving, dependable, or supportive?

Do you like yourself for other things you are good at or like to do, such as your job? Try to be very specific about what qualities you have.

Do you like any parts of your body, such as your hair, your eyes? Do you like your smile? Don't negate your whole body because you think you are fat.

Do you think you would be missed if you died? What would people miss about you? If you have children, what would they say about you? Would they only miss the services you provide for them, or are there personality traits and values that have had an impact on them? Would they only miss the meals you cooked and the times you drove them around? What about missing your love, emotional support, sense of humor? What about the person you are and what you have taught them?

What would your spouse miss about you? Could he or she easily replace you? Why did your spouse pick you to marry? If you don't know, ask.

You may think you have no impact on anyone. It is time to be more aware of how others experience you.

c. SELF-ESTEEM AND EATING

When you have low self-esteem, you tend to do things that will convince you and others that you are worthless. Keeping yourself out of shape is one way to do this. It helps you feel sorry for yourself and provides you with an excuse about why your life may not be the way you want. You must like yourself before you can give up overeating and the fat it causes.

You eat when your self-esteem is low because —

(a) you want to be fat and get sympathy from others.

(b) you feel unloved and eat to fill the void, or

(c) you want to use the food as a reward for feeling bad.

Your motivation may be good, but the results are bad. You eat to cope with your unhappiness about yourself, but you end up hating yourself for overeating or for getting fat. As a result, your self-esteem is lowered. Clearly, it would be more productive to find some other way to deal with your poor self-image.

In Exercise #14, check the old messages you believe, then read the truth about them, and begin to tell yourself the appropriate new messages.

EXERCISE #14
MESSAGES ABOUT SELF-ESTEEM

OLD MESSAGE	TRUTH	NEW MESSAGE
☐I can't like myself fat. I will like myself when I lose weight.	Your self-worth is based on more than weight. Old feelings make you envious of anyone who is thinner than you no matter how thin you get.	I like myself for me. I accept myself as I am. I want to lose weight to improve my appearance.
☐I can't like myself as a compulsive eater. It means I have no control.	You eat to cope with stress. You can learn other ways. You are human, and so you are not perfect. You must allow yourself to be whatever you are.	I will do what I can to find new ways to deal with stress. I accept myself as I am until then.
☐I think I am not all right because that is what others told me.	Others react to you based on their own feelings of imperfection. They are not always making objective evaluations. You know deep down when they are wrong about you.	I am O.K. because I am me. I trust my own evaluation of myself. If I am judged unfairly, I can object.
☐I must live up to what others expect of me to be a good person.	What others expect may have more to do with them than you. You must see yourself as a separate person, and let them cope with the real you.	I must be myself in order to love myself.
☐I must not praise myself.	When you put yourself down, you think it will prevent others from doing so. Actually, others think more negatively about you when you give them the idea to do so.	I owe it to myself to praise myself. I cannot wait for others to do so.
☐If people really knew me, they would not love me.	People will accept you if you are open about who you are, and if you respect yourself.	I am O.K. as I am. I can respect myself when I am truly me.

d. WORKING TOWARD POSITIVE CHANGE

Here are some things you can do to feel better about yourself:

(a) Praise yourself without making a judgment and without thinking that what you did was too trivial. Give yourself recognition for anything, no matter how small.

(b) Do what you do well. Give yourself opportunities to succeed where you have a talent or skill. This includes choice of career, hobbies, and courses. You will feel better about yourself when you have success.

(c) Accept your limitations. If possible, avoid situations you know mean failure. Allow yourself to be less than the best and to be good only at some things, not everything.

(d) Assert your rights. Let no one control you. Say "no" when you want to.

(e) Express your feelings, especially your anger and your desires. Make no judgment about them. All feelings are allowed.

(f) Become independent. Make your own decisions, and do things your way. Trust your intuition more than the opinions of others.

(g) Be good to yourself. Take care of your emotional and physical needs. Take a rest or a vacation, phone a friend, eat healthy foods. Love yourself enough to stop eating compulsively and to give yourself what you really want instead of the food.

Find something to praise yourself for every day. It can be for doing something well, having an insight, making a decision, expressing a feeling, or even for not doing something self-destructive. Make no judgments, and don't look for perfection. For one week, record your self-praise in Exercise #15.

EXERCISE #15
SELF-PRAISE

DAY	I PRAISED MYSELF TODAY FOR:
Monday	
Tuesday	
Wednesday	
Thursday	
Friday	
Saturday	
Sunday	

7

BODY IMAGE

If you feel fat, you probably let that feeling affect every aspect of your life. A negative body image leads to low self-esteem, which causes you to refuse to change your lifestyle, avoid social contacts, not look for a job, or whatever you say you would do if you were thin.

But what is "too" fat? The issue of looking fat, or of body image, is different from the issue of the physical difficulties of being overweight. Body image cannot be measured against the possible physical symptoms of high blood pressure, shortness of breath, or hypoglycemia, all of which may occur in an overweight person. Rather, body image is measured against arbitrary standards set by society, which change from time to time and place to place. For example, when the artist Peter Paul Rubens was alive (1577–1640), he painted large, robust women. Their rounded, flowing curves were thought beautiful at the time.

Among cultures that value eating and fatness as an indication of love and enjoyment of life, thinness is regarded as a sign of starvation or sickness.

In North America today, the emphasis is on thinness. Fashion models wear tight jeans and dresses that show their boyish, lean bodies. Diet books are best sellers, and diet centers are everywhere. Exercise and good nutrition are stressed in the media.

We live in a society where food is fairly inexpensive and quite plentiful. Ironically, while magazines display skinny models as the ideal figure, they fill their pages with tantalizing food ads. The messages are mixed: eat, eat, eat, but stay thin.

a. DEVELOPING AN IMAGE YOU CAN LIVE WITH

How do you decide if you are fat or thin? Is it a number on the scale? Is it clothing size? Is it your body measurements? Is it what or how much you eat? Fatness and thinness are relative. You may be fatter than some people, but you are also thinner than others. If you have labelled yourself fat, it doesn't matter what your size is. Your label for yourself may be very different from the one others give to you.

If you feel too fat, ask yourself, "Too fat for what?" Are you too fat to be healthy for long? Or to feel fit? These are legitimate reasons to lose weight. But if you feel too fat to fit into a size 10 or to wear jeans, or to be liked, you are applying damaging standards to your self-image.

Remember, if you believe you are going to turn from a shy, inhibited person into a ravishing free spirit just be shedding some weight, you will be disappointed. You will feel better about your appearance, but you cannot completely change your personality. Becoming thin does not alter a negative self-image. Many formerly fat people still have low self-esteem.

In Exercise #16, indicate what you like and what you dislike about your body. Try to find as many likes as dislikes. The things you like don't have to be perfect.

EXERCISE #16
BODY AWARENESS

	I LIKE:	I DISLIKE:
Eyes		
Hair		
Nose		
Mouth		
Arms		
Legs		
Hips		
Skin		
Feet		
Waist		
Hands		
Posture		
Teeth		

After doing this exercise, you may realize that you don't really hate your whole body. Do you appreciate your smile? Your hair? Your complexion? Do you like the shape of your hands or your hips or your legs? If you do, you need to keep in mind that no matter what you weigh, the basic shape of those parts of your body does not change. If you have broad shoulders or narrow hips, they will always be that way in proportion to the rest of your body.

Stop generalizing about your body as a whole. Enjoy the parts that you have always admired; try to lose weight on the parts that are obscured by some excess flesh. The human form is beautiful, and the only thing extra weight does is to blur it.

Few bodies are in true proportion, so try not to berate your body if it isn't one of them.

In Exercise #17, check the old messages you believe, then read the truth about them, and begin to tell yourself the appropriate new messages.

EXERCISE #17
MESSAGES ABOUT BEING FAT

OLD MESSAGE	TRUTH	NEW MESSAGE
☐My happiness depends on my losing weight.	Losing weight may make you feel better about your appearance, and you will be more sociable. It won't solve all your problems. By staying fat, you blame the fat and avoid dealing with anything else.	I want to improve my appearance by losing weight. It is up to me to take care of other problems I have.
☐Everyone sees my fat and so thinks less of me.	People are not that interested in your appearance and probably don't think you are as fat as you think. They relate to who you are, not what you look like.	I am the only one who cares what I look like.
☐My fat prevents me from getting a job, a lover, a friend.	There may be some prejudice about fat people, but there are many large people who are successful. The fat may be an excuse to keep you from doing what scares you.	My fat is my excuse. If I lose weight, I can still avoid those things that scare me or say no to people.
☐I need my fat to protect me from getting hurt.	If you are afraid of closeness, you would keep people away even if you were thin. If they stay away while you are fat, it is not the fat that keeps them away, but rather your unfriendliness.	I can get as close to others as I choose. I do not need my fat to keep others away.
☐My fat is not the real me.	You are your body, feelings, thoughts, impulses. You present the whole package to others.	My appearance is part of the real me.
☐If I am loved when fat, I know it is for the real me.	When you are thin, you are still presenting a whole person to which others are responding.	I owe it to myself to be the best me there is, including my appearance.

b. BODY IMAGE AND SEXUALITY

Your attitudes about sex and sexuality were developed in your early training at home. Perhaps your mother or father warned you about sex, so you grew up fearful of it. Perhaps your parents or church told you that sex before marriage was immoral and dirty. Whatever the messages were, they will affect how you feel about your own sexuality now.

Did you have a conflict with the attitudes taught to you as a child? Did you feel guilty about getting pleasure from sex? Some people interpret their childhood message about sex as: "I must not enjoy sex" and then as "I must not enjoy anything I do impulsively." Sometimes, this results in the need for secrecy in all pleasure, which can trigger secretive, compulsive eating.

You may have had some early negative experiences with sex that have made you uncomfortable with your sexual feelings or have led you to suppress them.

What are your attitudes now about sex, and about your role as a male or female? Where did those ideas come from? Do you want to change any of them?

Do Exercise #18 to help you think about your sexuality.

EXERCISE #18
SEXUALITY PROFILE

Complete the sentences below with one or more of these words: *passionate, inhibited, passive, aggressive, shy, modest, affectionate, nurturing, playful, innovative, provocative, conventional, prudish.*

1. To be feminine is to be _____ .

2. To be masculine is to be _____ .

3. To be sexy is to be _____ .

4. My father was _____ .

5. My mother was _____ .

6. I am _____ .

7. If I were thinner, I would be _____ .

8. If I were more sexual, then _____ .

Very often, uncomfortableness about sexuality is at the root of a compulsive eater's difficulties. Staying fat is one way to avoid the problems of dealing with your attractiveness and sexuality. Are you afraid of being too attractive? Some women fear they will be pursued by too many men if they are. What they really are afraid of is their inability to say no.

Are you afraid that if you were very attractive, others would be jealous? Often, this is a reflection of your need to please everyone.

Some people worry that if they are attractive they will never know if others want to be with them because of their looks or their personalities. If they stay fat and have friends, they are comforted, knowing their personalities are what attracts people.

When you worry about these things, staying fat is your protection. If you are afraid to be thin, you keep yourself fat by overeating. You may go on diets and lose weight, but always go off the diet when your weight reaches a certain point. You may use your weight as an excuse for not socializing.

You will be able to lose weight when, emotionally, you no longer need the fat to —

- keep you from having to say no to sex
- keep you from being promiscuous
- keep your mate from feeling threatened
- keep others from being jealous
- ensure you are wanted for the real you
- keep you from being rejected
- provide you with an excuse for a poor social life

Your inhibitions and your fears prevent you from having a fuller sexual life. You probably are not as fat as you think you are, but you use your fat as an excuse.

You can become more assertive and turn sex down, if you want, no matter what you weigh. You can then have sex in your life or not, as you wish. When you keep yourself as unattractive as possible, you limit the possibilities.

In Exercise #19, check the old messages you believe, then read the truth about them, and begin to tell yourself the appropriate new messages.

c. HOW YOU APPEAR TO OTHERS

How you appear to others is affected by many things: the clothes you wear, their style and color, your expression, your manner. Each of these things makes a non-verbal statement about you that may speak louder than words.

EXERCISE #19
MESSAGES ABOUT SEXUALITY

OLD MESSAGE	TRUTH	NEW MESSAGE
☐If I am sexual, I will be promiscuous.	You will always do only what you really want to do. Your upbringing would not allow otherwise.	I can trust myself to do only what I want to do.
☐I cannot say no to sex because I will hurt my partner.	You have the right to decide what to do with your body. Your partner must learn to cope with your saying no.	I can be honest and say what I want.
☐If I am sexual, I will be treated as a sex object.	You are only treated as a sex object when you let someone use your body without your consent.	I do not want to deprive myself of my sexuality. I can still set the limits.
☐My spouse will be threatened if I am sexy.	Your spouse will be pleased that others find you attractive, as long as he or she is sure of your feelings.	I can be the best I am and enjoy a better relationship with my spouse.
(For women) ☐I must not make sexual advances to men.	You are entitled to your impulses.	I am equal to men.
☐I must not be a threat to other women.	You may not get their approval if you are, but you will feel good about yourself if you are all you can be.	I cannot worry about what others think. I must be all I can be. I do not need to be loved by everyone.

The colors you wear can tell something about your personality. Warm clothes give a friendlier, less reserved message than cool ones. Pale colors may make you fade into the background, while bright ones say you are a person to be reckoned with. Black may make you look slimmer, but it may also make you look ghastly if it is wrong for your complexion, or it may indicate you are depressed.

What does the style of your clothes say about you? Do your clothes hide or enhance your shape? Even a thin person can look heavier in clothes that do not fit well. Are your clothes tailored? Frilly? Sexy? Each style makes a statement about who you are. What do you want to say with your clothes? Do you want to look unique? Do you want to blend into the background? You put on a costume when you get dressed, and it defines your role. Do you look very different when you go out than when you go to work?

Remember that your outward appearance, the one you present to the world through your clothes, your hairstyle, and your accessories, reflects your inner feelings, ideas, and fantasies.

Would you dress differently if you were thinner? Would you wear clothes that made you more noticeable? Probably you would not, because if you are shy, you will be shy at any weight. It is time to become more comfortable about your uniqueness, and let that be reflected in your dress. Your clothes can be a suit of armor to hide you, or they can enhance your best features. Your outward appearance is unlikely to change unless you have changed inside as well.

Do Exercise #20 to understand what sort of appearance you present to the world. Would you like to change anything? You don't have to wait until you lose weight.

EXERCISE #20
APPEARANCE CHECKLIST

Select the items that apply most often:

I choose clothes that are:

____tailored   ____sporty   ____frilly

____casual   ____off-beat   ____chic

I prefer this because _____.

The colors I most frequently wear are:

____pastel   ____warm   ____earthy

____dark   ____cool   ____bright

If I were thin, I would wear _____.

I wear my hair:

____long   ____curly   ____dyed

____short   ____straight   ____natural

                ____coiffed

8

MAKING CHANGES

If you have read this far in this book, you realize there are things in your life that you want to change — destructive things that make you unhappy. But change involves the unknown, and if you assume it will be worse than what you are doing, you will not easily put your present behavior aside. Like many people you may be afraid of change.

a. BECOMING COMFORTABLE ABOUT CHANGE

The problem with making no changes and "playing it safe" is that you stifle your needs. You may also find that your life is boring because it is repetitious and predictable; you learn nothing new about yourself (which only happens when you have new experiences); and you get stuck with decisions you have made, even when you are sorry you made them.

The healthy part of you wants growth, change, happiness, and the best for you. It wants to get out of situations that are destructive and into those that satisfy your needs. But the unhealthy part of you is too afraid of change, expects disaster to occur, or is waiting for things to improve by themselves.

So the two parts of you are in conflict, one side seeing the benefits of change and the other seeing the problems. It is easier to let the unhealthy part take over. You have to work to let the healthy part have priority. To see what your two sides are saying about change, do Exercise #21.

Many of your fears about making changes and pursuing what you want are based on old messages that are not accurate. In Exercise #22, check the old messages you believe, then read the truth about them, and begin to tell yourself the appropriate new messages.

EXERCISE #21
MAKING CHANGES

Write down the benefits and problems for you of making the following changes:

1. Being more independent:

    The benefits are _____ .

    The problems are _____ .

2. Being more assertive:

    The benefits are _____ .

    The problems are _____ .

3. Being thinner:

    The benefits are _____ .

    The problems are _____ .

4. Being more responsible

    The benefits are _____ .

    The problems are _____ .

Example: The benefits of being independent are increased self-esteem and freedom. The problems are loneliness and being a threat to others.

EXERCISE #22
MESSAGES ABOUT CHANGE

OLD MESSAGE	TRUTH	NEW MESSAGE
☐When I make a decision, I must stick to it.	You may be afraid of the unexpected that happens when you change your mind. You will enjoy the freedom that comes with it.	I have the right to change my mind, and I can cope with the results.
☐I have to structure my life so every moment is planned. Then I am safe from the unknown.	A rigid life is boring. You can learn to cope with the unknown.	I cannot control the future, and I will enjoy my life if I do not try to.
☐If I make any change in my behavior, I will go wild with it before I can stop.	Change happens slowly. You do not lose old inhibitions easily.	I can change at my own pace.
☐Getting thin guarantees good changes.	Thinness only changes your appearance. The rest you have to work on.	My weight is not responsible for anything else in my life.
☐Others will not be able to cope with any changes I make, so I better not make them.	If others can't cope, they may need professional help. You have to do what makes you feel good about you.	I will change whatever makes me feel good about me, as long as it does not hurt others.
☐Change is too scary. It is better to stay stuck.	Staying stuck means you are trapped and playing it safe. It does not give you a chance to experience much.	When you make a change, you feel more in control.

In order to become more comfortable with the idea of introducing changes in your life, you can start by changing things in a small way in order to add variety to your life. Here are some examples:

- Buy and serve a food you have never had before.
- Eat something different for breakfast.
- Serve and eat meals at new times.
- Try a new restaurant.
- Change your hair color or style.
- Buy a new color of clothing.
- Try a new activity, craft, or sport.
- Travel to a new place.
- Meet new people.
- Drive a new route to work.
- Read a new kind of book.

Part of making a change involves making a decision. Many factors enter into making that decision:

- Your upbringing, which influences you about what you *should* do, and which may be the opposite of what you *want* to do
- Your rational mind, with which you weigh all the consequences of your decision
- Other people, who may or may not approve of your decision
- Your ability to withstand criticism from those who don't approve
- Your "gut feeling" — your intuition — that tells you what is right for you

You can use your conscious mind to solve problems by processing all the information you have. But your final decision has to be based on what you intuitively know. If you go against what feels right, you will compensate in some way, like eating compulsively.

As a child, you, like most children, were probably able to react intuitively. Even without much knowledge about the world, you had feelings about places and people, such as which were safe, which were friendly, and which you could not trust. No one could fool you. You just *knew* who was lying and who was sincere.

As you grew up, you were taught to "look before you leap," to analyze everything. So you lost your intuitive ability because you stopped trusting it.

It is important to get back to using it. It makes you less dependent on the judgment of others and makes you feel in charge of your life. You are capable of making decisions if only you trust your intuitive wisdom. When you do that, change will be easier for you.

Use the worksheet in Exercise #23 to chart the changes you have already made and those you hope to make.

EXERCISE #23
CHANGE PROGRESS

1. I have changed these things about eating:

   • _____

   • _____

   • _____

   • _____

2. I have changed these things in my life:

   • _____

   • _____

   • _____

   • _____

3. I would like to make these additional changes:

   • _____

   • _____

   • _____

   • _____

4. What stops me is:

   • _____

   • _____

   • _____

   • _____

b. FEAR OF SUCCESS

Success means many different things to many different people. There is professional success, which involves recognition through a job promotion or salary increase or gaining a reputation in a particular field. There is emotional success, which means gaining insight and changing behavior that results in happiness and fulfillment. There is success at improving your skill in some task, such as mastering typing. There is success at achieving your goal, such as losing weight.

If it were just a simple matter of doing what you always do, without change, you would have constant success. Unfortunately, you may never succeed because of your fear of change. To risk changing and being successful means to risk failure as well.

But perhaps you not only fear failure, you fear success. If you have a task to complete that may lead to a major change in your life, you may find yourself putting it off. It may be the thesis that leads to a degree, the business deal that leads to a promotion, the application that leads to a job interview. Behind procrastination is often a fear of success.

Do Exercise #24 to see what stops you from being more successful. If possible, first record the entire exercise on a cassette tape and then play it back for yourself. Otherwise, just read one section at a time and follow the instructions given.

EXERCISE #24
CHANGE FANTASY

1. Sit comfortably in a chair. Shut out everything, close your eyes. Feel enormous. You are just a blob of fat, so heavy that you cannot move. You cannot get up from the chair. It is too much of an effort. Since you will never be thinner, you will have to stay in the chair from now on. See how this makes you feel. Is there anything you enjoy about this idea? When you are ready, open your eyes. Write your answers to the following questions.

    • Did you find this fantasy depressing? _____

    • Did you have the urge to make a change, to get up? _____

    • Do you try to do so in your life, or are you stuck in a rut? _____

    • Are you too paralyzed to move? _____

- Did you enjoy anything in this fantasy? _____

- Did you feel relieved to have an excuse not to make changes?

  _____

- Did that mean no chance to fail, so you felt safe? _____

When you do nothing, you take no risks. So doing nothing to change your life may be the easier choice.

2. Now close your eyes again, and see yourself overweight. Ahead of you is a door. If you open it, you can go to a world where whatever you want is waiting. Get up and open the door and go into this new world. See what is there and how you feel. Then open your eyes.

- What was behind the door? _____

- Who was there? _____

- What happened? _____

Perhaps you saw a world filled with happy people. Perhaps they were children because you want to return to an earlier time in your life that was without responsibility. Even if your childhood was not a happy one, you can have a fantasy about the way you wish it was. You may not like being an adult.

Perhaps you saw yourself behind the door as a success in some way, and in reality you avoid pursuing your talents. You do not want to face possible rejection, but you also miss out on possible recognition. Being overweight may just be your excuse for not doing what scares you.

One woman saw herself behind the door as a famous artist and thin. In reality, she avoids exhibiting her work because she is afraid of rejection. She keeps herself overweight to have an excuse for not showing her work, and she assumes it would be different if she were thinner.

- What is stopping you from going through the door? _____

  _____

- Do you have to be fat to protect yourself from going there? ____

  _____

If you have fears about making a change, give yourself permission to wait. Or make the change slowly. You may think the only change you can make is a drastic one, like getting a divorce, when you could make a gradual one, like going to a counselor or separating temporarily.

You may have preferred the first fantasy because you felt safer than in the second, which involved change. You may not want to try out your fantasies, fearing they may work out differently in real life and be proven impossible. Perhaps, then, your fantasies are based on exaggerated expectations of yourself. When you can make a fantasy less extreme, you are more likely to pursue your goals and make the necessary change.

You may avoid change because of negative messages that are not based on reality. In Exercise #25, check the old messages you believe, then read the truth about them, and begin to tell yourself the new messages.

EXERCISE #25
MESSAGES ABOUT SUCCESS

OLD MESSAGE	TRUTH	NEW MESSAGE
☐ If I lose weight, I will be expected to keep it off.	You (not others) have this expectation of yourself. The present is more important than the past. Only those in the public eye, like actors or sports figures, need to be concerned with past performances.	What I do today is more important than what I did yesterday. I can lose weight, and if I gain it back, I can decide what I want to do.
☐ If I can't diet perfectly, I might as well not try.	You can never be perfect at anything. You have to accept failure as part of life, and give yourself credit for any success. When there is failure, you have to begin again.	If I break my diet, I can begin again.
☐ If I tried to succeed, I would be the best. I just can't get started.	By not starting, you can believe you are perfect and not have to deal with failure. You must learn to accept your imperfections.	I can try to succeed, and if I don't, I can begin again. I need not do anything perfectly.

☐ I can get more attention from being a failure. Being a success means being a threat to others.	Some people are threatened by success, but it is more important to be what you can admire.	I have to do what makes me feel good about myself rather than worry about others.
☐ I am afraid of failing if I try anything new.	Failing usually means doing something less than perfectly. Not doing it at all is worse than doing your best, which may not be perfect.	I can be less than perfect and still be a success.

c. DEALING WITH PERFECTIONISM

When you set goals for yourself that are too high, you are doomed to failure and disappointment. You measure success as reaching those goals, and anything less as worthless. You then experience low self-esteem and depression.

You need to learn to credit yourself for your effort, whether you attain your goals or not. Constant frustration can affect your health and your interest in making a future effort. When your standards are more realistic, you can succeed more often.

This is not to say that you must not try to do your best. But your best may be less than you have decided it should be — less than perfect.

Compulsive eaters commonly believe that if they cannot do something perfectly, it is better not to do it at all. So, they deviate from their diets or give up all together.

You must learn to accept yourself as imperfect, to allow yourself to make mistakes, and to go on from there. If you overeat at one meal, you can make up for it by eating less later that day or the next one. You don't have to give up all you have gained.

When you can love your *real* self, you will not stop loving yourself just because you are not perfect all the time in every way.

You can become less of a perfectionist by doing the following:

- Try to see the inbetweens, instead of seeing everything in extremes.
- Live in the present, instead of in the future or the past.
- Set lower standards for yourself and for others.
- Allow yourself and others to make mistakes.
- Give yourself credit for what you do.
- Get rid of "always" and "never," replace them with "sometimes" and "usually" in your thoughts and conversations.

69

9

EATING WITHOUT GUILT

a. PLEASURE AND EATING

When you diet, you stop eating some of the foods you love. You replace these with foods you feel neutral about or dislike. Or you limit the amount you can eat of foods that give you pleasure. When you get fed up with this deprivation, you binge. That is why diets don't work for compulsive eaters, who feel it is wrong to enjoy eating. The way to eat less is to increase your pleasure in other areas. What these will be depends on your interests. If you have believed that having pleasure means being a hedonist, you have denied yourself a great deal. Life must be a balance.

Ideally, you should allow yourself all the foods you enjoy, while adding activities and experiences that give you other pleasures. In time, you will be able to focus more on other things, so you will eat less. And, when you do eat, you will enjoy the experience and not feel guilty.

Fill out the questionnaire in Exercise #26 before reading further.

Did you find it difficult to list 20 things you love to do? If so, perhaps you overlooked some obvious ones, such as taking a walk or a nap. Did you include eating, or do you have too much guilt when you eat to enjoy it?

An activity you enjoy does not have to be spectacular. If you really love to talk on the phone, that should be on your list. Do not place a value judgment on any item you wish to include.

Do you usually do what you enjoy, or have you found that most of the things you have listed are things you never get around to doing? Do you really lack the time, or do you avoid pleasure because of negative connotations, such as selfishness, that you attach to it. A life without pleasure is dull, and this leads you to use food to provide what is missing.

Think about what you do each day, and consider whether some of your time could be better spent. If you work, do you enjoy your job? You spend so much of your day at work that you should consider changing jobs if you get no pleasure from the one you have.

If you do not work, and you have a family, do you do mostly meaningless chores all day? Do you spend longer than necessary at the supermarket? Do you do the laundry when you have children

EXERCISE #26
PLEASURE QUESTIONNAIRE

The things that give me pleasure, that I most love to do are:

1. _____   11. _____

2. _____   12. _____

3. _____   13. _____

4. _____   14. _____

5. _____   15. _____

6. _____   16. _____

7. _____   17. _____

8. _____   18. _____

9. _____   19. _____

10. _____ 20. _____

The ones I usually get to do are (put a check next to them).

The high point of every day is when _____,

because _____.

The low point of every day is when _____,

because _____.

I see from this list that I need to _____

_____.

who are old enough to do it? Do you make extra trips when you could combine your errands? Do you waste a lot of time?

See how your eating fits in with what you do in a day. Are you eating at times because:

- You don't know what else to do.
- You want to avoid doing chores that wait for you.
- You want to have some pleasure.

Look at your pleasures list again. Is there some way you could do *all* the activities you listed in the immediate future? As a way to get started, do Exercise #27.

EXERCISE #27
PLEASURE ACTIVITIES

Do something you love to do every day. Write down what it is and what effect it has, if any, on your eating (amount, food, time of day).

DAY	PLEASURE ACTIVITY	EFFECT ON EATING
Monday		
Tuesday		
Wednesday		
Thursday		
Friday		
Saturday		
Sunday		

b. BOREDOM

Do you sometimes eat because you are bored and want to pass the time? You cannot think of anything you want to do and looking at the pleasures list you made doesn't help because you are even bored with those things.

Often, boredom is just hiding real feelings. If you live alone, you may have a lot of time on your hands, and you may think you are bored. It is possible that a lot of that feeling is really anger, which you have repressed. So you eat, and tell yourself it is because you are bored.

You may say you are bored because you have a moment with nothing scheduled. Try to allow yourself to just do nothing. Do you look at that as a waste of time? Try to see it as a chance to free yourself from too much routine or from too many distractions in your environment. Sit quietly, relax, and unwind. This kind of doing nothing is actually doing something.

c. SELF-ASSESSMENT

It is important to know how you have grown since you began reading this book. You have to give yourself credit for all the insights you have gained, for any changes you have made in behavior, for being interested enough in helping yourself to do the exercises.

If you are dissatisfied with yourself because you have not completely eliminated self-destructive behaviors or because you have not become someone you hoped you would be, you are still being a perfectionist. You have to eliminate preconceived notions about yourself, and take each day at a time.

The only comparisons you should ever make are to what you did yesterday. If today you are doing something a little differently, in a more positive way, you have made progress. Tomorrow may go up or down, but most likely your progress will be upward. That is, if you don't jeopardize the progress you have made by being overly critical or too impatient.

Exercise #28 will help you see how you have progressed. It is in two parts: eating behavior and other life areas. Put a check next to every thing you usually do now. Usually does not mean always. It is unrealistic to expect that you will not have times when you revert to old behavior, especially when there is considerable stress.

The items left after you have checked everything you can indicate those behaviors you still need to work on. Circle them on the sheet, and check them off as you continue to make progress in the weeks and months to come.

EXERCISE #28
PROGRESS CHECKLIST

Check those items that apply to what you *usually* do now.

EATING
____I eat without feeling guilty.
____I eat only when I am hungry.
____I stop eating when I am full.
____I only eat at the table.
____I skip meals when I want to.
____I have reduced my sugar intake.
____I only eat what I like.
____I eat slower than before.
____I can throw out food.
____I allow myself occasional treats.

____I can say no to an offer of food.
____When I do binge, I know why.
____I eat a good breakfast.

BODY
____I accept my body.
____I weigh myself occasionally.
____I dress to look my best.
____I enjoy my sexuality.
____I care about my health.
____I do regular exercise.

LIFE AREAS
____I accept my behavior.
____I praise myself.
____I give myself treats other than food.
____I can say no to others.
____I look for love instead of pity.
____I live in the present.
____I express my anger.
____I am independent.
____I make my own decisions

____I set reachable goals.
____I take responsibility for what I do.
____I can make mistakes.
____I can change my mind.
____I express positive feelings.
____I can wait without panic.
____I can admit mistakes.
____I apologize less frequently.
____I see the good in my life.
____I can be spontaneous.

d. WHAT NOW?

You can feel good about all you have learned and about the progress you have made.

This is not the time to quit. Go back to the chapters in the book that apply to the issues you have still not resolved. Read them and do the exercises again. Your answers will not necessarily be the same. It would be good to compare them now that you have more insight.

Read as many books on the Recommended Reading list as you can (see page 77). The more you know, the more your grow. Keep notes, so when you find helpful passages, you can refer to them again.

You might be ready now to join a support group to work on your eating, your self-image, and your relationships.

If you think it would be helpful, join a group set up for weight loss. Just be sure you are not treated like someone who cannot decide anything and told by someone else what to eat. Don't join a group where you will be berated for not losing weight. You need support and insight, not criticism.

Above all, be patient. You have a lifetime ahead of you in which to learn and grow. Keep working on it.

Good luck to you!

RECOMMENDED READING

a. COMPULSIVE EATING

Arenson, Gloria. *How to Stop Playing the Weighting Game.* New York: St. Martin's Press, 1981.

_____. *Binge Eating.* New York: Rawson Associates, 1984.

Bockar, Joyce A. *The Last Best Diet Book.* Briarcliff Manor, NY: Stein & Day, 1980.

Jordan, Henry A., Levitz, Leonard S., and Kimbrell, Gordon M. *Eating is Okay: A Radical Approach to Weight Loss.* Edited by Steve Gelman. New York: New American Library, Signet Books, 1978.

LeShan, Eda. *Winning the Losing Battle: Why I Will Never Be Fat Again.* New York: Bantam Books, 1981.

Marston, Albert R. *The Undiet: A Psychological Approach to Permanent Weight Control.* Englewood Cliffs, NJ: Prentice-Hall, Inc., 1983.

Millman, Marcia. *Such a Pretty Face: Being Fat in America.* New York: Berkley Publishing, 1982.

Orbach, Susie. *Fat is a Feminist Issue: The Anti-Diet Guide to Permanent Weight Loss.* New York: Berkley Books, 1979.

_____. *Fat is a Feminist Issue II: A Program to Conquer Compulsive Eating.* New York: Berkley Books, 1982.

Pearson, Leonard, and Pearson, Lillian. *The Psychologist's Eat Anything Diet Book.* New York: David McKay Co., Inc., Peter H. Wyden, Inc., 1973.

Ray, Sondra. *The Only Diet There Is.* Millbrae, CA: Celestial Arts Publishing Co., 1981.

Roth, Geneen. *Feeding the Hungry Heart.* New York: Bobbs-Merrill Co., Inc., 1982.

Schwartz, Bob. *Diets Don't Work!* rev. ed. Houston, TX: Breakthru Publishing, 1984.

Stern, Frances M., and Hoch, Ruth S. *Mind Trips to Help You Lose Weight.* New York: Berkley Publishing, Jove Publications, Inc., 1977.

Ter Heun, Pat, and Smith, Lynda. *Being Fat Has Nothing To Do With Food: A Handbook for the Yo-Yo-Dieter.* Millbrae, CA: Celestial Arts, 1981.

Wardell, Judy, and Austin, Barbara. *Thin Within: How To Eat and Live Like a Thin Person.* New York: Crown Publications, Inc., 1985.

Westin, Jeane E. *Break Out of Your Fat Cell: A Holistic Mind-Body Guide to Permanent Weight Loss*. Minneapolis, MN: CompCare Publications, 1979.

Wise, Jonathan K., and Wise, Susan K. *The Overeaters: Eating Styles and Personality*. New York: Human Sciences Press, Inc., 1979.

b. SELF DEVELOPMENT

Bach, Dr. George R., and Deutsch, Ronald M. *Stop! You're Driving Me Crazy*. New York: Berkley Publishing, 1985.

Browne, Harry. *How I Found Freedom in an Unfree World*. New York: Avon Books, 1974.

Bry, Adelaide, and Bair, Marjorie. *Directing the Movies of Your Mind: Visualization for Health and Insight*. New York: Harper & Row, 1978.

Dodson, Dr. Fitzhugh. *The You That Could Be*. New York: Pocket Books, 1977.

Dowling, Colette. *The Cinderella Complex: Women's Hidden Fear of Independence*. New York: Pocket Books, 1982.

Dyer, Wayne. *Pulling Your Own Strings*. New York: Avon Books, 1979.

————. *Your Erroneous Zones*. New York: Avon Books, 1981.

Fensterheim, Herbert, and Baer, Jean. *Don't Say Yes When You Want to Say No*. New York: Dell, 1975.

Glasser, William. *Positive Addiction*. New York: Harper & Row, 1976.

Greenburg, Dan, and Jacobs, Marcia. *How to Make Yourself Miserable*. New York: Random House, 1966.

Huxley, Laura. *You Are Not the Target*. Los Angeles: J. P. Tarcher, Inc., 1985.

Jacobs, Dorri. *Priorities: How to Stay Young and Keep Growing*. New York: Franklin Watts, Inc., 1978.

————. *Change: How to Live With, Manage, Create and Enjoy It*. New York: Programs on Change, 1981.

Keen, Sam. *What to Do When You're Bored and Blue*. New York: Putnam Publishing Group, Wideview Books, 1981.

Lair, Jess. *I Ain't Much Baby, But I'm All I've Got*. New York: Fawcett Book Group, 1978.

Leatz, Christine Ann. *Unwinding*. Englewood Cliffs, NJ: Prentice Hall, Inc., 1981.

Lowen, Alexander. *Pleasure: A Creative Approach to Life*. New York: Penguin, 1975.

Newman, Mildred, and Berkowitz, Bernard. *How to Be Your Own Best Friend*. With Jean Owen. New York: Ballantine, 1974.

Pietsch, William V. *Human Be-Ing: How to Have a Creative Relationship Instead of a Power Struggle*. New York: New American Library, 1984.

Viscott, David S. *Feel Free*. New York: David McKay Co., Inc., Peter H. Wyden, Inc., 1971.

c. NUTRITION AND COOKING

Bricklin, Mark. *Lose Weight Naturally: The No-Diet, No Willpower Plan from Prevention Magazine*. Emmaus, PA: Rodale Press, 1979.

Brody, Jane. *Jane Brody's Nutrition Book*. New York: Bantam Books, 1982.

Claiborne, Craig, and Franey, Pierre. *Craig Claiborne's Gourmet Diet*. New York: Ballantine, 1981.

Gibbons, Barbara. *The Slim Gourmet Cookbook*. New York: Harper & Row, 1976.

Lappe, Frances M. *Diet for a Small Planet*. New York: Ballantine, 1975.

TITLES AVAILABLE
FROM
SELF-COUNSEL PRESS

PERSONAL HELP TITLES

AIDS TO INDEPENDENCE
This book is a comprehensive catalogue of products available to help the disabled and elderly function effectively and live a full and satisfying life. Black and white photographs illustrate the aids.

BETWEEN THE SEXES
Whether you've been together two years or twenty, this book is designed to help you break through the cycles of frustration or anger in your relationship and work toward a positive lifestyle.

FAMILY TIES THAT BIND
This book explains a proven approach for dealing with the complications of family relationships and establishing more positive directions in your life.

MANAGING STRESS
This book covers general health and well-being, personal planning skills, communication skills, quieting, autogenic methods, and progressive relaxation training. Each technique helps take the worry out of worrying.

A PARENTS' GUIDE TO DAY CARE
This comprehensive consumer's guide to child care alternatives shows parents how to inform themselves about the choices and how to make day care a positive experience.

RETIREMENT GUIDE
For those who are unprepared, retirement is both a shock and a disappointment. This guide gives counsel on how to prepare for a healthy, happy, and financially secure retirement.
Editions available for Canada and U.S. West Coast only. See order form.

TAKING CARE
Practical advice for anyone in a prolonged situation of caretaking an adult relative or spouse.

WORKING COUPLES
Being a working couple doesn't have to mean having constant conflict in your life. This practical guide takes a straightforward approach to the issues involved when both people in a relationship are working outside the home.

CAREER DEVELOPMENT AND REFERENCE

THE HANDY GUIDE TO ABBREVIATIONS AND ACRONYMS FOR THE AUTOMATED OFFICE
Over 7000 abbreviations and acronyms commonly used in the fields of computers, law, business, and medicine are defined.

ASKING QUESTIONS
Entertaining, informative guide to the art of the interview based on the experience of dozens of well-known interviewers.

BETTER BOOK FOR GETTING HIRED
The focus of this book is on the importance of the resume. You may be short changing yourself by not giving the prospective employer an accurate picture of your talents.
Available in Canada only.

EDITING YOUR NEWSLETTER
For anyone who edits a regular newsletter this book discusses how to establish the goals of your newsletter, how to distribute it, and how to produce a quality item with a limited budget.
Available in Canada only.

GETTING ELECTED
Here is a guide to electioneering at the grass-roots level. If you're interested in running for office for the local schoolboard, city hall, or town council, this guide will help lead you to success.
Available in Canada only.

KEYBOARDING FOR KIDS
Here is a new system for teaching children keyboarding skills to use on a typewriter or computer set up in 10 lessons, requiring two 10-15 minute practice sessions each day. Part 2 provides advanced skills for older children.

LEARN TO TYPE FAST
This new system of learning how to type, which you can learn in five hours, teaches you the keys in relation to your fingers, rather than the keyboard.

THE UPPER LEFT-HAND CORNER
This book is for writers looking to the growing markets in the upper left-hand corner of North America. It lists hundreds of publishers and contains a wealth of information to aid anyone in the business of writing.

CANADIAN
ORDER FORM
SELF-COUNSEL SERIES

04/86

NATIONAL TITLES:

_____	Abbreviations & Acronyms	5.95
_____	Aids to Independence	7.95
_____	Asking Questions	11.95
_____	Assertiveness for Managers	8.95
_____	Basic Accounting	5.95
_____	Be a Better Manager	7.95
_____	Best Ways	5.50
_____	Better Book for Getting Hired	9.95
_____	Between the Sexes	8.95
_____	Business Guide to Effective Speaking	6.95
_____	Business Guide to Telephone Systems	7.95
_____	Business Writing Workbook	9.95
_____	Buying (and Selling) a Small Business	6.95
_____	Changing Your Name in Canada	3.50
_____	Civil Rights	8.95
_____	Collection Techniques for the Small Business	4.95
_____	Complete Guide to Being Your Own Home Contractor	19.95
_____	Credit, Debt, and Bankruptcy	5.95
_____	Criminal Procedure in Canada	14.95
_____	Design Your Own Logo	9.95
_____	Drinking and Driving	4.50
_____	Editing Your Newsletter	14.95
_____	Entrepreneur's Self-Assessment Guide	9.95
_____	Exporting	12.50
_____	Family Ties That Bind	7.95
_____	Federal Incorporation and Business Guide	14.95
_____	Financial Control for the Small Business	6.95
_____	Financial Freedom on $5 A Day	7.95
_____	For Sale By Owner	4.95
_____	Franchising in Canada	6.50
_____	Fundraising	5.50
_____	Getting Elected	8.95
_____	Getting Sales	14.95
_____	Getting Started	11.95
_____	How to Advertise	7.95
_____	How You Too Can Make a Million . . . In the Mail Order Business	8.95
_____	Immigrating to Canada	14.95
_____	Immigrating to the U.S.A.	14.95
_____	Importing	21.95
_____	Insuring Business Risks	3.50
_____	Keyboarding for Kids	7.95
_____	Landlording in Canada	12.95
_____	Learn to Type Fast	9.95
_____	Managing Your Office Records and Files	14.95
_____	Managing Stress	7.95
_____	Media Law Handbook	6.50
_____	Medical Law Handbook	6.95
_____	Mike Grenby's Money Book	5.50
_____	Mike Grenby's Tax Tips	6.95
_____	Mortgage and Foreclosure Handbook	6.95
_____	Musician's Handbook	7.95
_____	Parents' Guide to Day Care	5.95
_____	Photography & The Law	)5
_____	Practical Guide to Financial Management	J5
_____	Ready-to-Use Business Forms	9.95
_____	Resort Condos	4.50
_____	Retirement Guide for Canadians	9.95
_____	Start and Run a Profitable Beauty Salon	14.95
_____	Start and Run a Profitable Consulting Business	12.95
_____	Start and Run a Profitable Craft Business	10.95
_____	Start and Run a Profitable Home Typing Business	9.95
_____	Start and Run a Profitable Restaurant	10.95
_____	Start and Run a Profitable Retail Business	11.95
_____	Start and Run a Profitable Video Store	10.95
_____	Starting a Successful Business in Canada	12.95
_____	Taking Care	7.95
_____	Tax Law Handbook	12.95
_____	Tax Shelters	6.95
_____	Trusts and Trust Companies	3.95
_____	Upper Left-Hand Corner	10.95
_____	Using the Access to Information Act	5.95
_____	Word Processing	8.95
_____	Working Couples	5.50
_____	Write Right!	(Cloth) 5.95 / (Paper) 5.50

PROVINCIAL TITLES:

Please indicate which provincial edition is required.

Consumer Book
☐B.C. 7.95   ☐Ontario 6.95

Divorce Guide
☐B.C. 12.95   ☐Alberta   ☐Ontario   ☐Man./Sask.

Employee/Employer Rights
☐B.C. 6.95   ☐Alberta 6.95   ☐Ontario 6.95

Fight That Ticket
☐B.C. 5.95   ☐Ontario 3.95

Incorporation Guide
☐B.C. 14.95   ☐Alberta 14.95   ☐Ontario 14.95   ☐Man./Sask. 12.95

Landlord/Tenant Rights
☐B.C. 7.95   ☐Alberta 6.95   ☐Ontario 7.95

Marriage & Family Law
☐B.C. 7.95   ☐Alberta 5.95   ☐Ontario 7.95

Probate Guide
☐B.C. 12.95   ☐Alberta 9.95   ☐Ontario 11.95

Real Estate Guide
☐B.C. 7.95   ☐Alberta 7.95   ☐Ontario 7.95

Small Claims Court Guide
☐B.C. 6.95   ☐Alberta 7.50   ☐Ontario 5.95

Wills
☐B.C. 5.95   ☐Alberta 5.95   ☐Ontario 5.50

Wills/Probate Procedure
☐Man./Sask 5.95

PACKAGED FORMS:

Divorce
☐B.C. 12.95   ☐Alberta 12.95   ☐Ontario   ☐Man.   ☐Sask.

Incorporation
☐B.C. 12.95   ☐Alberta 12.95   ☐Ontario 14.95

☐Man. 14.95   ☐Sask. 14.95   ☐Federal 7.95

☐Minute Books 16.50

Probate
☐B.C. Administration 14.95   ☐B.C. Probate 14.95   ☐Alberta 14.95   ☐Ontario 15.50

Sell Your Own Home
☐B.C. 4.95   ☐Alberta 4.95   ☐Ontario 4.95

☐Rental Form Kit (B.C., Alberta, Ontario, Sask.)   5.95

☐Have You Made Your Will?   5.95

☐If You Love Me Put It In Writing   Contract Kit   9.95

☐If You Leave Me Put It In Writing   B.C. Separation Agreement Kit   14.95

NOTE: All prices subject to change without notice.

Books are available in book and department stores, or use the order form below.

Please enclose cheque or money order (plus sales tax where applicable) or give us your MasterCard or Visa Number (please include validation and expiry date.)

(PLEASE PRINT)

Name _____

Address _____

City _____ Postal Code _____

☐Visa/☐MasterCard Number _____

Validation Date _____ Expiry Date _____

If order is under $20.00, add $1.00 for postage and handling.

Please send orders to:

INTERNATIONAL SELF-COUNSEL PRESS LTD.   ☐Check here for free catalogue.
306 West 25th Street
North Vancouver, British Columbia
V7N 2G1

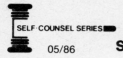

AMERICAN
ORDER FORM
SELF-COUNSEL SERIES

NATIONAL TITLES

____	Abbreviations & Acronyms	$5.95
____	Aids to Independence	11.95
____	Asking Questions	7.95
____	Assertiveness for Managers	8.95
____	Basic Accounting for the Small Business	5.95
____	Be a Better Manager	7.95
____	Between the Sexes	8.95
____	Business Guide to Effective Speaking	6.95
____	Business Guide to Telephone Systems	7.95
____	Business Writing Workbook	9.95
____	Buying (and Selling) a Small Business	6.95
____	Collection Techniques for the Small Business	4.95
____	Design Your Own Logo	9.95
____	Entrepreneur's Self-Assessment Guide	9.95
____	Exporting from the U.S.A.	12.95
____	Family Ties that Bind	7.95
____	Financial Control for the Small Business	5.50
____	Financial Freedom on $5 a Day	7.95
____	Franchising in the U.S.	5.95
____	Fundraising for Non-Profit Groups	5.50
____	Getting Sales	14.95
____	How You Too Can Make a Million in the Mail Order Business	8.95
____	Immigrating to Canada	14.95
____	Immigrating to the U.S.A.	14.95
____	Keyboarding for Kids	7.95
____	Learn to Type Fast	9.95
____	Managing Stress	7.95
____	Musician's Handbook	7.95
____	Parent's Guide to Day Care	5.95
____	Photography and the Law	7.95
____	Practical Guide to Financial Management	5.95
____	Ready-to-Use Business Forms	9.95
____	Resort Condos & Time Sharing	4.50
____	Retirement in the Pacific Northwest	4.95
____	Start and Run a Profitable Beauty Salon	14.95
____	Start and Run a Profitable Consulting Business	12.95
____	Start and Run a Profitable Craft Business	10.95
____	Start and Run a Profitable Home Typing Business	9.95
____	Start and Run a Profitable Restaurant	10.95
____	Start and Run a Profitable Retail Store	11.95
____	Start and Run a Profitable Video Store	10.95
____	Starting a Successful Business on West Coast	12.95
____	Taking Care	7.95
____	Upper Left-Hand Corner	10.95
____	Word Processing	8.95
____	Working Couples	5.50

STATE TITLES
Please indicate which state edition is required.

____ Divorce Guide
☐ Washington (with forms) 12.95 ☐ Oregon 11.95